The Walker's Literary Companion

THE
WALKER'S
LITERARY
COMPANION

Edited by

Roger Gilbert   Jeffrey Robinson   Anne Wallace

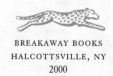

BREAKAWAY BOOKS
HALCOTTSVILLE, NY
2000

The Walker's Literary Companion

ISBN: 1-891369-19-9

LIBRARY OF CONGRESS CATALOG CARD NUMBER: 99-85883

Published by Breakaway Books
P. O. Box 24
Halcottsville, NY 12438
(800) 548-4348
www.breakawaybooks.com

Distributed by Consortium

FIRST EDITION

CONTENTS

PREFACE

Going out for a long walk, the nineteenth-century novelist and essayist Robert Louis Stevenson would bring with him the classic English walking essay, William Hazlitt's "On Going a Journey" (1821), about which he claimed, passionately if dogmatically, it is "so good that there should be a tax levied on all who have not read it." Imagine being so taken with an essay on walking! But history, at least of the past two hundred years, reveals that walkers have loved to read about their passion; and—given the perennial market for magazine essays and fictions, poems, and novels either describing a walk or set on a walk—that nonwalking readers also like to imagine life occurring on the path or pavement.

The three editors have in common a love of walking and love of the literature of walking. We are all university scholars who have written books on literature and walking, and through this last connection have come to know one another. The mutually infectious nature of the subject and our dedication to it led to the present volume. To this end we have walked the streets of Manhattan and around the Central Park Reservoir, huddled in a Chicago hotel room, and tramped the bluffs on the northern California coast, culling from memory our favorite walking pieces from the great collective wellspring of human writing.

We have composed our anthology for both pedestrian and nonpedestrian readers. Is there a person alive, except for the physically disabled, who is not a walker? Everyone walks, but we address those who love walking, either on the ground or in the imagination. When about a hundred years ago he compiled *The Lore of the Wanderer: An Open-Air Anthology,* a small plain blue-covered book one could put in a back pocket, George Goodchild—in perhaps the first of a substantial cluster of such collections—caught the spirit of our end-of-this-century volume: a book (a companion) to be taken with you; or, if you cannot get out for a walk, you can read one at home.

There are, however, important differences between Goodchild's collection and ours. By "Open-Air" he meant the air of the countryside far from the polluting enclosures of the city. By insisting upon walking as a rural pleasure, Goodchild blinded his readers to the rich array of urban walking literature. We include many walks in nature (and even "Sunday Walks in the Suburbs") but also want to open up the world of the urban walker's imagination. Goodchild, moreover, cultivated a kind of men's club version of walking pleasure: gentle and gentile, leisurely, contemplative, healthy, and pure. But city walking reminds us that walking is the right or necessity of all classes of persons and can, as much as enlisting one's sense of protected leisure, occasion vulnerabilities. Walking can be dangerous, particularly for women alone. Sometimes we walk simply to get from one point to another, with no thought of particular pleasure. And there are those who walk because they can't afford any more rapid means of transportation. Yet writers of the urban walk, finally, catch the extraordinary vitality and variety of the city and at times make us believe that as a species we can be our best there.

Just as different kinds and intentions of walking abound, so the literature of walking comes to us in many forms, styles, and genres. Indeed, walking literature beautifully subsumes to itself the range of formal possibilities in literature. Our anthology thus includes: passages from novels and long poems, essays, and lyric poems composed in classic forms but also in experimental contemporary ones. Walking becomes an analogy to the act of writing and to the movement and rhythms of poetry and prose, a proof of the more general truth that energy and movement belong fundamentally to good writing and visionary and creative thinking. Moreover, writers from around the world and from ancient times to the present have chosen to represent their experience of the walk, which, together with the formal range, helps to comprise in this book a small window on the history of world literature. And while we have culled the majority of our selections from the past two hundred years (when walking has increased as a sport or pastime with a correspondent increase in literary representations of the walk) and from writers of the English language, we have by a smaller number of examples indicated the potential worldwide and worldhistorical interest of our subject.

Writers have found walking analogous to and a way of grounding other human activities such as talking and thinking and writing, a giving form to other, less physical domains of our being. Submersion in the following collection may lead one to propose that "the walk" models a well-lived life: one always in motion but at different speeds, moving forward but with circlings back and pauses along the way, encountering obstructions and bearing burdens and perhaps for a time overcoming both, immersing oneself in detail and then gaining perspectives, shifting from social to solitary occasions, growing in self-consciousness and knowledge and recovering innocence, becoming the "host" and being the "guest" and the "stranger," encountering those who embrace and those who reject your walking status, feeling isolated and feeling communal, witnessing the good and evil events of humankind. Walking literature, at a lesser or greater remove, hearkens to the magnificent and possibly universal metaphor: "Life is a journey."

Our anthology does not claim to lead the reader to a conclusive understanding of what a walk is; like a walk itself, this book has only an imposed end, determined here by the necessary limits of publication. As every step on a walk brings, potentially, an unexpected view or experience, so every piece in our collection takes the reader on an unexpected path. Neither do we claim comprehensiveness. To us walking literature seems nearly infinite: for every piece we discover, we have come to expect that two others lie waiting to be found. Everyone seems to know some walking piece. Having put together this anthology, we have had to reject at least another containing yet as many different items. What you have before you are the current favorites of your editors.

A book can be like a walk. How could we best emulate in *The Walker's Literary Companion* the walking experience? All the standard methods of organization seemed to us too predictive: chronological by author, thematic, generic. We decided to present the materials alphabetically by title: you never know where you will step next. Several years ago a precedent for this came to our attention: *The Rattle Bag,* an anthology of lyric poetry edited by Seamus Heaney and the late Ted Hughes (Faber and Faber). We have been encouraged in our effort by the continued popularity of this book—for general readers and students. The happiest reader of our book may, of course, disregard organization altogether and strike out in unanticipated directions across the meadow of these pages. At times, however, one wishes to read together all the selections upon one thematic grouping (e.g. night walks, rural walks, urban walks): for this we provide an index at the back.

   Roger Gilbert   *Jeffrey Robinson*   *Anne Wallace*

Dorothy Wordsworth
FROM THE ALFOXDEN JOURNAL

Alfoxden, January 20th, 1798. —The green paths down the hillsides are channels for streams. The young wheat is streaked by silver lines of water running between the ridges, the sheep are gathered together on the slopes. After the wet dark days, the country seems more populous. It peoples itself in the sunbeams. The garden, mimic of spring, is gay with flowers. The purple-starred hepatica spreads itself in the sun, and the clustering snow-drops put forth their white heads, at first upright, ribbed with green, and like a rosebud when completely opened, hanging their heads downwards, but slowly lengthening their slender stems. The slanting woods of an unvarying brown, showing the light through the thin net-work of their upper boughs. Upon the highest ridge of that round hill covered with planted oaks, the shafts of the trees show in the light like the columns of a ruin.

January 21st. Walked on the hill-tops—a warm day. Sate under the firs in the park. The tops of the beeches of a brown-red, or crimson. Those oaks, fanned by the sea breeze, thick with feathery sea-green moss, as a grove not stripped of its leaves. Moss cups more proper than acorns for fairy goblets.

January 22nd. —Walked through the wood to Holford. The ivy twisting round the oaks like bristled serpents. The day cold—a warm shelter in the hollies, capriciously bearing berries. Query: Are the male and female flowers on separate trees?

January 23rd. —Bright sunshine, went out at 3 o'clock. The sea perfectly calm blue, streaked with deeper colour by the clouds, and tongues or points of sand; on our return of a gloomy red. The sun gone down. The crescent moon, Jupiter, and Venus. The sound of the sea distinctly heard on the tops of the hills, which we could never hear in summer. We attribute this partly to the bareness of the trees, but chiefly to the absence of the singing of birds, the hum of insects, that noiseless noise which lives in the summer air. The villages marked out by beautiful beds of smoke. The turf fading into the mountain road. The scarlet flowers of the moss.

January 24th. —Walked between half-past three and half-past five. The evening cold and clear. The sea of a sober grey, streaked by the deeper grey clouds, The half dead sound of the near sheep-bell, in the hollow of the sloping coombe, exquisitely soothing.

January 25th. —Went to Poole's after tea. The sky spread over with one continuous cloud, whitened by the light of the moon, which, though her dim shape was seen, did not throw forth so strong a light as to chequer the earth with shadows. At once the clouds seemed to cleave asunder, and left her in the centre of a black-blue vault. She sailed along, followed by multitudes of stars, small, and bright, and sharp. Their brightness seemed concentrated, (half-moon).

January 26th. —Walked upon the hill-tops; followed the sheep tracks till we overlooked the larger coombe. Sat in the sunshine. The distant sheep-bells, the sound of the stream; the woodman winding along the half-marked road with his laden pony; locks of wool still spangled with the dewdrops; the blue-grey sea, shaded with immense masses of cloud, not streaked; the sheep glittering in the sunshine. Returned through the wood. The trees skirting the wood, being exposed more directly to the action of the sea breeze, stripped of the net-work of their upper boughs, which are stiff and erect, like black skeletons; the ground streaked with the red berries of the holly. Set forward before two o'clock. Returned a little after four.

January 27th. —Walked from seven o'clock till half-past eight. Upon the whole an uninteresting evening. Only once while we were in the wood the moon burst through the invisible veil which enveloped her, the shadows of the oaks blackened, and their lines became more strongly marked. The withered leaves were coloured with a deeper yellow, a brighter gloss spotted the hollies; again her form became dimmer; the sky flat, unmarked by distances, a white thin cloud. The manufacturer's dog makes a strange, uncouth howl, which it continues many minutes after there is no noise near it but that of the brook. It howls at the murmur of the village stream.

January 28th. —Walked only to the mill.

January 29th. —A very stormy day. William walked to the top of the hill to see the sea. Nothing distinguishable but a heavy blackness. An immense bough riven from one of the fir trees.

January 30th. —William called me into the garden to observe a singular appearance about the moon. A perfect rainbow, within the bow one star, only of colours more vivid. The semicircle soon became a complete circle, and in the course of three or four minutes the whole faded away. Walked to the blacksmith's and the baker's; an uninteresting evening.

January 31st. —Set forward to Stowey at half-past five. A violent storm in the wood; sheltered under the hollies. When we left home the moon immensely large, the sky scattered over with clouds. These soon closed in, contracting the dimensions of the moon without concealing her. The sound of the pattering shower, and the gusts of wind, very grand. Left the wood when nothing remained of the storm but the driving wind, and a few scattering drops of rain. Presently all clear, Venus first showing herself between the struggling clouds; afterwards Jupiter appeared. The hawthorn hedges, black and pointed, glittering with millions of diamond drops; the hollies shining with broader patches of light. The road to the village of Holford glittered like another stream. On our return, the wind high—a violent storm of hail and rain at the Castle of Comfort. All the Heavens seemed in one perpetual motion when the rain ceased; the moon appearing, now half veiled, and now retired behind heavy clouds, the stars still moving, the roads very dirty.

February 1st. —About two hours before dinner, set forward towards Mr. Bartholomew's. The wind blew so keen in our faces that we felt ourselves inclined to seek the covert of the wood. There we had a warm shelter, gathered a burthen of large rotten boughs blown down by the wind of the preceding night. The sun shone clear, but all at once a heavy blackness hung over the sea. The trees almost roared, and the ground seemed in motion with the multitudes of dancing leaves, which made a rustling sound, distinct from that of the trees. Still the asses pastured in quietness under the hollies, undisturbed by these forerunners of the storm. The wind beat furiously against us as we returned. Full moon. She rose in uncommon majesty over the sea, slowly ascending through the clouds. Sat with the window open an hour in the moonlight.

February 2nd. —Walked through the wood, and on to the Downs before dinner; a warm pleasant air. The sun shone, but was often obscured by straggling clouds. The redbreasts made a ceaseless song in the woods. The wind rose very high in the evening. The room smoked so that we were obliged to quit it. Young lambs in a green pasture in the Coombe, thick legs, large heads, black staring eyes.

February 3rd. —A mild morning, the windows open at breakfast, the red-breasts singing in the garden. Walked with Coleridge over the hills. The sea at first obscured by vapour; that vapour afterwards slid in one mighty mass along the seashore; the islands and one point of land clear beyond it. The distant country (which was purple in the clear full air), overhung by straggling clouds that sailed over it, appeared like the darker clouds, which are often seen at a great distance apparently motionless, while the nearer ones pass quickly over them, driven by the lower winds. I never saw such a union of earth, sky, and sea. The clouds beneath our feet spread themselves to the water, and the clouds of the sky almost joined them. Gathered sticks in the wood; a perfect stillness. The redbreasts sang upon the leafless boughs. Of a great number of sheep in the field, only one standing. Returned to dinner at five o'clock. The moonlight still and warm as a summer's night at nine o'clock

February 4th. —Walked a great part of the way to Stowey with Coleridge. The morning warm and sunny. The young lasses seen on the hill-tops, in the villages and roads, in their summer holiday clothes—pink petticoats and blue. Mothers with their children in arms, and the little ones that could just walk, tottering by their side. Midges or small flies spinning in the sunshine; the songs of the lark and redbreast; daisies upon the turf; the hazels in blossom; honeysuckles budding. I saw one solitary strawberry flower under a hedge. The furze gay with blossom. The moss rubbed from the pailings by the sheep, that leave locks of wool, and the red marks with which they are spotted, upon the wood.

Philip Levine
ASK FOR NOTHING

Instead walk alone in the evening
heading out of town toward the fields
asleep under a darkening sky;
the dust risen from your steps transforms
itself into a golden rain fallen
earthward as a gift from no known god.
The plane trees along the canal bank,
the few valley poplars, hold their breath
as you cross the wooden bridge that leads
nowhere you haven't been, for this walk
repeats itself once or more a day.
That is why in the distance you see
beyond the first ridge of low hills
where nothing ever grows, men and women
astride mules, on horseback, some even
on foot, all the lost family you
never prayed to see, praying to see you,
chanting and singing to bring the moon
down into the last of the sunlight.
Behind you the windows of the town
blink on and off, the houses close down;
ahead the voices fade like music
over deep water, and then are gone;
even the sudden, tumbling finches
have fled into smoke, and the one road
whitened in moonlight leads everywhere.

Elizabeth Barrett Browning
FROM AURORA LEIGH

from FIRST BOOK.

Whoever lives true life will love true love.
I learnt to love that England. Very oft,
Before the day was born, or otherwise
Through secret windings of the afternoons,
I threw my hunters off and plunged myself
Among the deep hills, as a hunted stag
Will take the waters, shivering with the fear
And passion of the course. And when at last
Escaped, —so many a green slope built on slope
Betwixt me and the enemy's house behind,
I dared to rest, or wander, —like a rest
Made sweeter for the step upon the grass,—
And view the ground's most gentle dimplement,
(As if God's finger touched but did not press
In making England!), such an up and down
Of verdure,—nothing too much up or down,
A ripple of land; such little hills, the sky
Can stoop to tenderly and the wheatfields climb;
Such nooks of valleys lined with orchises,
Fed full of noises by invisible streams;
And open pastures, where you scarcely tell
White daisies from white dew,—at intervals
The mythic oaks and elm-trees standing out
Self-poised upon their prodigy of shade,—
I thought my father's land was worthy too
Of being my Shakespeare's. . . .

from SECOND BOOK.

Times followed one another. Came a morn
I stood upon the brink of twenty years,
And looked before and after, as I stood
Woman and artist,—either incomplete,
Both credulous of completion. There I held
The whole creation in my little cup,
And smiled with thirsty lips before I drank,
'Good health to you and me, sweet neighbour mine,
And all these peoples.'
                              I was glad, that day;
The June was in me, with its multitudes
Of nightingales all singing in the dark,
And rosebuds reddening where the calyx split.
I felt so young, so strong, so sure of God!
So glad, I could not choose be very wise!
And, old at twenty, was inclined to pull
My childhood backward in a childish jest
To see the face of 't once more, and farewell!
In which fantastic mood I bounded forth
At early morning,—would not wait so long
As even to snatch my bonnet by the strings,
But, brushing a green trail across the lawn
With my gown in the dew, took will and way
Among the acacias of the shrubberies,
To fly my fancies in the open air
And keep my birthday. . . .

John Hollander
BREAD-AND-BUTTER!

Walking together for so many years
They could hold hand in hand and still avoid
What a jackhammer or a dog had done
To or on the sidewalk—such was the supple
Touch they kept in, such the ample closeness
That marked their every way of walking by
The way (and sitting in their house and lying
Down and rising up, for all that, as well)

And what they would pass by on either side—
On each one's side—dissolved into the air,
The general air, of the phase or stage of things
They and their local walk were moving through
Until it seemed that they could not be said
To share the walk they took so much as that
The walk itself, a tall, responsible
Adult, went between them, holding both their hands

Until they happened on the unexpected
Obstacle—and whether it had leapt up
As an expanded stumbling-block too massy
And oddly-formed merely to trip over,
Or cried out silently and suddenly
In an abyss, all hands parted, they passed

He to the left	She rightward then with *Bread*
Around it, saying *Bread*	*And Butter!* and
And Butter! out	Of touch and loss of touch;

Of phase and finally out
    Of contact with
Some mass of palpable,
    Immediate
Souvenir then, and yet
    Avoiding that
Abyss of memory
    The phrase's taste
Upon his uttering tongue
    Could open up.
By then his hands no more
    Could even feel
Anticipations of
    A touch regained;
These two could not be read
    As from above,
Say, as "the two of them":
    Looking across
The separation now
    Had made no sense
For some time now in fact
    Or fiction too.
Only our love of closures
    Keeps us longing
For bridges, tunnels, hands
    But there was no
Common pathway ahead
    no *You that way* . . .
Ending some comedy
    as holding out
Against time, holding out
    Both hands and hope

Of childhood that
Had lingered with her long,
    The phrase she spoke
Itself spoke; but by then
    The time for hands
Laughingly to rejoin
    Was gone. The gap
Between them now was all
    The making of
Their walk itself; the way
    She took, the way
She had been taking now
    Was not just hers,
Let alone part of theirs,
    But merely all
The way there was. The cut
    Lines on the sidewalk
Between the concrete squares
    And which the games
Of childhood cut so deep
    Were not the same
There on the other side.
    Only our lust
For soft connections still
    Keeps us in quest
Of some clear syntax here.
    Both, neither, said:
We this way—a confirmed
    Deferral or
Contemporary sort
    Of difference
As if it were a word

Enough, though, of such literal narratives:
They had buttered their bread and eaten it.

Now distances shall not allow our straining
Eyes to track their faint courses any more
Where only the limitations of some page
Had made their ways seem to run parallel,
And only death would lay them lower than
The concrete actualities they walked
And leave them holding hands again with dust.

Robert Browning
BY THE FIRE-SIDE

I

How well I know what I mean to do
   When the long dark autumn-evenings come;
And where, my soul, is thy pleasant hue?
   With the music of all thy voices, dumb
In life's November too!

II

I shall be found by the fire, suppose,
   O'er a great wise book as beseemeth age,
While the shutters flap as the cross-wind blows
   And I turn the page, and I turn the page,
Not verse now, only prose!

III

Till the young ones whisper, finger on lip,
   'There he is at it, deep in Greek:
'Now then, or never, out we slip
   'To cut from the hazels by the creek
'A mainmast for our ship!'

IV

I shall be at it indeed, my friends
   Greek puts already on either side
Such a branch-work forth as soon extends
   To a vista opening far and wide,
And I pass out where it ends.

V

The outside-frame, like your hazel-trees:
   But the inside-archway widens fast,
And a rarer sort succeeds to these,
   And we slope to Italy at last
And youth, by green degrees.

VI

I follow wherever I am led,
   Knowing so well the leader's hand:
Oh woman-country, wooed not wed,
   Loved all the more by earth's male-lands,
Laid to their hearts instead!

VII

Look at the ruined chapel again
   Half-way up in the Alpine gorge!
Is that a tower, I point you plain,
   Or is it a mill, or an iron-forge
Breaks solitude in vain?

VIII

A turn, and we stand in the heart of things;
   The woods are round us, heaped and dim;
From slab to slab how it slips and springs,
   The thread of water single and slim,
Through the ravage some torrent brings!

IX

Does it feed the little lake below?
   That speck of white just on its marge
Is Pella; see, in the evening glow,
   How sharp the silver spear-heads charge
When Alp meets heaven in snow!

X

On our other side is the straight-up rock;
   And a path is kept 'twixt the gorge and it
By boulder-stones where lichens mock
   The marks on a moth, and small ferns fit
Their teeth to the polished block.

XI

Oh the sense of the yellow mountain flowers,
   And thorny balls, each three in one,
The chestnuts throw on our path in showers!
   For the drop of the woodland fruit's begun,
These early November hours,

XII

That crimson the creeper's leaf across
  Like a splash of blood, intense, abrupt,
O'er a shield else gold from rim to boss,
  And lay it for show on the fairy-cupped
Elf-needled mat of moss,

XIII

By the rose-flesh mushrooms, undivulged
  Last evening—nay, in to-day's first dew
Yon sudden coral nipple bulged,
  Where a freaked fawn-coloured flaky crew
Of toadstools peep indulged.

XIV

And yonder, at foot of the fronting ridge
  That takes the turn to a range beyond,
Is the chapel reached by the one-arched bridge
  Where the water is stopped in a stagnant pond
Danced over by the midge.

XV

The chapel and bridge are of stone alike,
  Blackish-grey and mostly wet;
Cut hemp-stalks steep in the narrow dyke.
  See here again, how the lichens fret
And the roots of the ivy strike! . . .

XX

And all day long a bird sings there,
  And a stray sheep drinks at the pond at times;
The place is silent and aware;
  It has had its scenes, its joys and crimes,
But that is its own affair.

XXI

My perfect wife, my Leonor,
  Oh heart, my own, oh eyes, mine too,
Whom else could I dare look backward for,
  With whom beside should I dare pursue
The path grey heads abhor?

XXII

For it leads to a crag's sheer edge with them;
　　Youth, flowery all the way, there stops—
Not they; age threatens and they contemn,
　　Till they reach the gulf wherein youth drops,
One inch from life's safe hem!

XXIII

With me, youth led . . . I will speak now,
　　No longer watch you as you sit
Reading by fire-light, that great brow
　　And the spirit-small hand propping it,
Mutely, my heart knows how—

XXIV

When, if I think but deep enough,
　　You are wont to answer, prompt as rhyme;
And you, too, find without rebuff
　　Response your soul seeks many a time
Piercing its fine flesh-stuff.

XXV

My own, confirm me! If I tread
　　This path back, is it not in pride
To think how little I dreamed it led
　　To an age so blest that, by its side,
Youth seems the waste instead? . . .

XXX

Come back with me to the first of all,
　　Let us lean and love it over again,
Let us now forget and now recall,
　　Break the rosary in a pearly rain,
And gather what we let fall!

XXXI

What did I say?—that a small bird sings
　　All day long, save when a brown pair
Of hawks from the wood float with wide wings
　　Strained to a bell: 'gainst noon-day glare
You count the streaks and rings.

XXXII

But at afternoon or almost eve
    'T is better; then the silence grows
To that degree, you half believe
    It must get rid of what it knows,
Its bosom does so heave.

XXXIII

Hither we walked then, side by side,
    Arm in arm and cheek to cheek,
And still I questioned or replied,
    While my heart, convulsed to really speak,
Lay choking in its pride.

XXXIV

Silent the crumbling bridge we cross,
    And pity and praise the chapel sweet,
And care about the fresco's loss,
    And wish for our souls a like retreat,
And wonder at the moss.

XXXV

Stoop and kneel on the settle under,
    Look through the window's grated square:
Nothing to see! For fear of plunder,
    The cross is down and the altar bare,
As if thieves don't fear thunder.

XXXVI

We stoop and look in through the grate,
    See the little porch and rustic door,
Read duly the dead builder's date;
    Then cross the bridge that we crossed before,
Take the path again—but wait!

XXXVII

Oh moment, one and infinite!
    The water slips o'er stock and stone;
The West is tender, hardly bright:
    How grey at once is the evening grown—
One star, its chrysolite!

XXXVIII

We two stood there with never a third,
  But each by each, as each knew well:
The sights we saw and the sounds we heard,
  The lights and the shades made up a spell
Till the trouble grew and stirred.

XXXIX

Oh, the little more, and how much it is!
  And the little less, and what worlds away!
How a sound shall quicken content to bliss,
  Or a breath suspend the blood's best play,
And life be a proof of this!

XL

Had she willed it, still had stood the screen
  So slight, so sure, 'twixt my love and her:
I could fix her face with a guard between,
  And find her soul as when friends confer,
Friends—lovers that might have been.

XLI

For my heart had a touch of the woodland-time,
  Wanting to sleep now over its best.
Shake the whole tree in the summer-prime,
  But bring to the last leaf no such test!
'Hold the last fast!' runs the rhyme.

XLII

For a chance to make your little much,
  To gain a lover and lose a friend,
Venture the tree and a myriad such,
  When nothing you mar but the year can mend:
But a last leaf—fear to touch!

XLIII

Yet should it unfasten itself and fall
  Eddying down till it find your face
At some slight wind—best chance of all!
  Be your heart henceforth its dwelling-place
You trembled to forestall!

XLIV

Worth how well, those dark grey eyes,
  That hair so dark and dear, how worth
That a man should strive and agonize,
  And taste a veriest hell on earth
For the hope of such a prize!

XLV

You might have turned and tried a man,
  Set him a space to weary and wear,
And prove which suited more your plan,
  His best of hope or his worst despair,
Yet end as he began.

XLVI

But you spared me this, like the heart you are,
  And filled my empty heart at a word.
If two lives join, there is oft a scar,
  They are one and one, with a shadowy third;
One near one is too far.

XLVII

A moment after, and hands unseen
  Were hanging the night around us fast;
But we knew that a bar was broken between
  Life and life: we were mixed at last
In spite of the mortal screen.

XLVIII

The forests had done it; there they stood;
  We caught for a moment the powers at play:
They had mingled us so, for once and good,
  Their work was done—we might go or stay,
They relapsed to their ancient mood.

XLIX

How the world is made for each of us!
  How all we perceive and know in it
Tends to some moment's product thus,
  When a soul declares itself—to wit,
By its fruit, the thing it does!

L

Be hate that fruit or love that fruit,
   It forwards the general deed of man,
And each of the Many helps to recruit
   The life of the race by a general plan;
Each living his own, to boot.

LI

I am named and known by that moment's feat;
   There took my station and degree;
So grew my own small life complete,
   As nature obtained her best of me—
One born to love you, sweet!

LII

And to watch you sink by the fire-side now
   Back again, as you mutely sit
Musing by fire-light, that great brow
   And the spirit-small hand propping it,
Yonder, my heart knows how!

LIII

So, earth has gained by one man the more,
   And the gain of earth must be heaven's gain too;
And the whole is well worth thinking o'er
   When autumn comes: which I mean to do
One day, as I said before.

Oliver Goldsmith
A CITY NIGHT-PIECE

From Lien Chi Altangi, to Fum Hoam, first president of the Ceremonial Academy at Pekin, in China.

The clock just struck two, the expiring taper rises and sinks in the socket, the watchman forgets the hour in slumber, the laborious and the happy are at rest, and nothing wakes but meditation, guilt, revelry and despair. The drunkard once more fills the destroying bowl, the robber walks his midnight round, and the suicide lifts his guilty arm against his own sacred person.

Let me no longer waste the night over the page of antiquity, or the sallies of contemporary genius, but pursue the solitary walk, where vanity, ever changing, but a few hours past, walked before me, where she kept up the pageant, and now, like a froward child, seems hushed with her own importunities.

What a gloom hangs all around! the dying lamp feebly emits a yellow gleam, no sound is heard but of the chiming clock, or the distant watch-dog. All the bustle of human pride is forgotten, an hour like this may well display the emptiness of human vanity.

There will come a time when this temporary solitude may be made continual, and the city itself, like its inhabitants, fade away, and leave a desart in its room.

What cities, as great as this, have once triumph'd in existence, had their victories as great, joy as just, and as unbounded, and with short-sighted presumption, promised themselves immortality. Posterity can hardly trace the situation of some. The sorrowful traveller wanders over the awful ruins of others, and as he beholds, he learns wisdom, and feels the transience of every sublunary possession.

Here, he cries, stood their citadel, now grown over with weeds; there their senate-house, but now the haunt of every noxious reptile; temples and theatres stood here, now only an undistinguished heap of ruin. They are fallen, for luxury and avarice first made them feeble. The rewards of state were conferred on amusing, and not on useful members of society. Their riches and opulence invited the invaders, who, though at first repulsed, returned again, conquered by perseverance, and at last swept the defendants into undistinguished destruction.

How few appear in those streets, which but some few hours ago were crowded; and those who appear, now no longer wear their daily mask, nor attempt to hide their lewdness or their misery.

But who are those who make the streets their couch, and find a short repose from wretchedness at the doors of the opulent? These are strangers, wanderers, and orphans, whose circumstances are too humble to expect redress, and whose distresses are too great even for pity. Their wretchedness excites rather horror than pity. Some are without the covering even of rags, and others emaciated with disease; the world has disclaimed them; society turns its back upon their distress, and has given them up to nakedness and hunger. These poor shivering females, have once seen happier days, and been flattered into beauty. They have been prostituted to the gay luxurious villain, and are now turned out to meet the severity of winter. Perhaps now lying at the doors of their betrayers they sue to wretches whose hearts are insensible, or debauchees who may curse, but will not relieve them.

Why, why was I born a man, and yet see the sufferings of wretches I cannot relieve! Poor houseless creatures! the world will give you reproaches, but will not give you relief. The slightest misfortunes of the great, the most imaginary uneasinesses of the rich, are aggravated with all the power of eloquence, and held up to engage our attention and sympathetic sorrow. The poor weep unheeded, persecuted by every subordinate species of tyranny, and every law, which gives others security, becomes an enemy to them.

Why was this heart of mine formed with so much sensibility! or why was not my fortune adapted to its impulse! Tenderness, without a capacity of relieving, only makes the man who feels it more wretched than the object which sues for assistance. Adieu.

Richard Jefferies
CLEMATIS LANE

Wild clematis grew so thickly on one side of the narrow lane that the hedge seemed made of it. Trailing over the low bushes, the leaves hid the hawthorn and bramble, so that the hedge was covered with clematis leaf and flower. The innumerable pale flowers gave out a faint odour, and coloured the sides of the highway. Rising up the hazel rods and taller hawthorn, the tendrils hung downwards and suspended the flowers overhead. Across the field, where a hill rose and was dotted with bushes—those bushes, too, were concealed by clematis, and though the flowers were so pale, their numbers tinted the slope. A cropped nut-tree hedge, again, low, but five or six yards thick, was bound together by the bines of the same creeping plant, twisting in and out, and holding it together. No care or art could have led it over the branches in so graceful a manner; the lane was festooned for the triumphal progress of the waggons laden with corn. Here and there, on the dry bank over which the clematis projected like an eave, there stood tall campanulas, their blue bells as large as the fingerstall of a foxglove. The slender purple spires of the climbing vetch were lifted above the low bushes to which it clung; there were ferns deeper in the hedge, and yellow bedstraw by the gateways. A few blackberries were ripe, but the clematis seemed to have overcome the brambles, and spoilt their yield. Nuts, reddened at the tip, were visible on the higher hazel boughs; they were ripe, but difficult to get at.

Leaving the lane by a waggon track—a gipsy track through a copse—there were large bunches of pale-red berries hanging from the wayfaring trees, or wild viburnum, and green and red berries of bryony wreathed among the branches. The bryony leaves had turned, some were pale buff already. Among the many berries of autumn those of the wayfaring tree may be known by their flattened shape, as if the sides had been pressed in like a flask. The bushes were not high enough for shadow, and the harvest sun was hot between them. The track led past the foot of a steep headland of the Downs, which could not be left without an ascent. Dry and slippery, the short grass gave no hold to the feet, and it was necessary to step in the holes cut through the turf for the purpose. Pushed forward from the main line of the Downs, the buff headland projected into the Weald, as headlands on the southern side of the range project into the sea. Towards the summit the brow came out somewhat, and even the rude steps in the turf were not much assistance in climbing this almost perpendicular wall of sward. Above the brow the ascent became easy; these brows raised steeper than the general slope are often found on the higher hills. A circular entrenchment encloses the summit, but the rampart has much sunk, and is in places levelled. Here it was pleasant to look back upon the beech woods at the foot of the great Downs, and far over the endless fields of the Weald or plain. Thirty fields could be counted in succession, one after the other, like irregular chess-squares, some corn, some grass, and these only extended to the first undulation, where the woods hid the fields behind them. But beyond these, in reality, succeeded another series of fields to the second undulation, and still a third series to the farthest undulation visible. Yet farther there was a faint line of hills, a dark cloud-like bank in the extreme distance. To the right and to the left were similar views. Reapers were at work in the wheat below, but already much of the corn had been carried, and the hour of a threshing engine came up from the ricks. A woodpecker called loudly in the beech wood; a "wish-wish" in the air overhead was caused by the swift motion of a wood-pigeon passing from "holt" to "hurst," from copse to copse. On the dry short turf of the hill-top even the shadow of a swallow was visible as he flew but a few yards high.

In a little hollow where the rougher grasses grew longer a blue butterfly fluttered and could not get out. He was entangled with his own wings, he could not guide himself between the grass tops; his wings fluttered and carried him back again. The grass was like a net to him, and there he fluttered till the wind lifted him out, and gave him the freedom of the hills. One small green orchis stood in the grass, alone; the harebells were many. It is curious that, if gathered, in a few hours (if pressed between paper) they become a deeper blue than when growing. Another butterfly went over, large and velvety, flying head to the wind, but unable to make way against it, and so carried sidelong across the current. From the summit of the hill he drifted out into the air five hundred feet above the flowers of the plain. Perhaps it was a peacock; for there was a peacock-butterfly in Clematis Lane. The harebells swung, and the dry tips of the grass bent to the wind which came over the hills from the sea, but from which the sun had dried the sea-moisture, leaving it twice refined—once by the passage above a hundred miles of wave and foam and again by the grasses and the hills, which forced the current to a higher level, where the sunbeams dried it. Twice refined, the air was strong and pure, sweet like the scent of a flower. If the air at the sea-beach is good, that of the hills above the sea is at least twice as good, and twice as strengthening. It possesses all the virtue of the sea air without the moisture which ultimately loosens the joints, and seems to penetrate to the very nerves. Those who desire air and quick recovery should go to the hills, where the wind has a scent of the sunbeams.

In the short time since ascending the slope the definition of the view has changed. At first it was clear indeed, and no one would have supposed there was any mist. But now suddenly every hill stands out sharp and definite; the scattered hawthorn bushes are distinct; the hills look higher than before. From about the woods an impalpable bluish mistiness that was there just now has been blown away. The yellow squares of stubble—just cleared—far below are whiter and look drier. I think it is the air that tints everything. This fresh stratum now sweeping over has altered the appearance of the country and given me a new scene. The invisible air, as if charged with colour, has spread another tone broadly over the landscape. Omitting no detail, it has worked out afresh every little bough of the scattered hawthorn bushes, and made each twig distinct. It is the air that tints everything.

While I have been thinking, a flock of sheep has stolen quietly into the space enclosed by the entrenchment. With the iron head of his crook placed against his breast, and the handle aslant to the ground, the shepherd leans against it, and looks down upon the reapers. He is a young man, and has a bright, intelligent expression on his features. Alone with his sheep so many hours, he is glad of some one to talk to, and points out to me the various places in view. The copses that cover the slopes of the hills he calls "holts"; there are three or four within a short distance. His crook is not a Pyecombe crook (for the best crooks used to be made at Pyecombe, a little Down hamlet), but he has another, which was made from a Pyecombe pattern. The village craftsman, whose shepherd's crooks were sought for all along the South Downs, is no more, and he has left no one able to carry on his work. He had an apprentice, but the apprentice has taken to another craft, and cannot make crooks. The Pyecombe crook has a curve or semicircle, and then opens straight; the straight part starts at a tangent from the semicircle. How difficult it is to describe so simple a matter as a shepherd's crook! In some way or other this Pyecombe form is found more effective for capturing sheep, but it is not so easy to make. The crook he held in his hand opened with an elongated curve. It appeared very small beside the ordinary crooks; this, he said, was an advantage, as it would hold a lamb. Another he showed me had the ordinary hook; this was bought at Brighton. The curve was too big, and a sheep could get its leg out; besides which, the iron was soft, and when a sheep was caught the iron bent and enlarged, and so let the sheep go. The handles were of hazel: one handle was straight, smooth, and the best in appearance—but he said it was weak; the other handle, which was crooked and rough-looking, was twice as strong. They used hazel rods for handles—ash rods were apt to "fly," *i.e.* break.

Wages were now fifteen shillings a week. The "farm hands"—elsewhere labourers—had fifteen shillings a week, and paid one shilling and sixpence a week for their cottages. The new cottages that had been built were two shillings and sixpence a week. They liked the old cottages best, not only because they were cheaper, but because they had larger gardens attached. It seemed that the men were fairly satisfied with their earnings; just then, of course, they were receiving much more for harvest work, such as lying up after the reaping machine at seven shillings and sixpence per acre. Clothes were the heaviest item of expenditure, especially where there was a family and the children were not old enough to earn anything. Except that he said "wid" for with—"wid" this, instead of with this—he scarcely mispronounced a word, speaking as distinctly and expressing himself as clearly as any one could possibly do. The briskness of manner, quick apprehension, and directness of answer showed a well-trained mind. The Sussex shepherd on this lonely hill was quite the equal of any man in his rank of life, and superior in politeness to many who move in more civilised places. He left me to fetch some wattles, called flakes in other counties; a stronger sort of hurdles. Most of the reaping is now done by machine, still there were men cutting wheat by hand at the foot of the hill. They call their reaphooks swaphooks, or swophooks, and are of opinion that although the machine answers well and clears the ground quickly when the corn stands up, if it is beaten down the swaphook is preferable. The swaphook is the same as the fagging-hook of other districts. Every hawthorn bush now bears its red berries, or haws; these are called "hog-hazels." In the west they are called "peggles." "Sweel" is an odd Sussex word, meaning to singe linen. People who live towards the hills (which are near the coast) say that places farther inland are more "uperds"—up the country—up towards Tunbridge, for instance.

The grasshoppers sang merrily round me as I sat on the sward; the warm sun and cloudless sky and the dry turf pleased them. Though cloudless, the wind rendered the warmth pleasant, so that the sunbeams, from which there was no shade, were not oppressive. The grasshoppers sang, the wind swept through the grass and swung the harebells, the "drowsy hum" of the threshing engine rose up from the plain; the low slumberous melody of harvest time floated in the air. An hour had gone by imperceptibly before I descended the slope to Clematis Lane. Out in the stubble where the wheat had just been cut, down amongst the dry short stalks of straw, were the light-blue petals of the grey field veronica. Almost the very first of field flowers in the earliest days of spring, when the rain drives over the furrow, and hail may hap at any time, here it was blooming in the midst of the harvest. Two scenes could scarcely be more dissimilar than the wet and stormy hours of the early year, and the dry, hot time of harvest; the pale blue veronica, with one white petal, flourished in both, true and faithful. The gates beside the lane were not gates at all, but double draw-bars framed together, so that the gate did not open on a hinge, but had to be drawn out of the mortices. Looking over one of these grey and lichened draw-bars in a hazel hedge there were the shocks of wheat standing within the field, and on them a flock of rooks helping themselves freely.

Lower in the valley, where there was water, the tall willow-herbs stood up high as the hedges. On the banks of a pool water-plantains had sent up stalks a yard high, branched, and each branch bearing its three-petalled flower. In a copse near the stems of cow-parsnip stood quite seven feet, drawn up by the willow bushes—these great plants are some of the largest that grow in the country. Goatsbeard grew by the wayside; it is like the dandelion, but has dark spots in the centre of the disc, and the flower shuts at noon. The wild carrots were forming their "birds' nests"—so soon as the flowering is over the umbel closes into the shape of a cup or bird's nest. The flower of the wild carrot is white; it is made up of numerous small separate florets on an umbel, and in the centre of these tiny florets is a deep crimson one. Getting down towards the sea and the houses now I found a shrub of henbane by the dusty road, dusty itself, grey-green, and draggled; I call it a shrub, though a plant because of its shrub-like look. The flowers were over—they are a peculiar colour, dark and green veined and red, there is no exact term for it, but you may know the plant by the leaves, which, if crushed, smell like those of the black currant. This is one of the old English medicinal plants still in use. The figs were ripening fast in an orchard; the fig trees are frequently grown between apple trees, which shelter them, and some of the fruit was enclosed in muslin bags to protect it. The fig orchards along the coast suggest thoughts of Italy and the ancient Roman galleys which crossed the sea to the Sussex ports. There is a curious statement in a classic author, to the effect that a letter written by Julius Caesar, when in Britain, on the Kalends of September, reached Rome on the fourth day before the Kalends of October, showing how long a letter was being carried from the South Coast to the centre of Italy, nineteen centuries ago.

A. R. Ammons
CORSONS INLET

I went for a walk over the dunes again this morning
to the sea,
then turned right along
   the surf
                  rounded a naked headland
                  and returned

along the inlet shore:

it was muggy sunny, the wind from the sea steady and high,
crisp in the running sand,
      some breakthroughs of sun
   but after a bit

continuous overcast:

the walk liberating, I was released from forms,
from the perpendiculars,
      straight lines, blocks, boxes, binds
of thought
into the hues, shadings, rises, flowing bends and blends
         of sight:

                  I allow myself eddies of meaning:
yield to a direction of significance
running
like a stream through the geography of my work:
      you can find

in my sayings
                swerves of action
                like the inlet's cutting edge:
        there are dunes of motion,
organizations of grass, white sandy paths of remembrance
in the overall wandering of mirroring mind:

but Overall is beyond me: is the sum of these events
I cannot draw, the ledger I cannot keep, the accounting
beyond the account:

in nature there are few sharp lines: there are areas of
primrose
        more or less dispersed;
disorderly orders of bayberry; between the rows
of dunes,
irregular swamps of reeds,
though not reeds alone, but grass, bayberry, yarrow, all . . .
predominantly reeds:

I have reached no conclusions, have erected no boundaries,
shutting out and shutting in, separating inside
        from outside: I have
        drawn no lines:
        as

manifold events of sand
change the dune's shape that will not be the same shape
tomorrow,

so I am willing to go along, to accept
the becoming
thought, to stake off no beginnings or ends, establish
        no walls:

by transitions the land falls from grassy dunes to creek
to undercreek: but there are no lines, though
    change in that transition is clear
    as any sharpness: but "sharpness" spread out,
allowed to occur over a wider range
than mental lines can keep:

the moon was full last night: today, low tide was low:
black shoals of mussels exposed to the risk
of air
and, earlier, of sun,
waved in and out with the waterline, waterline inexact,
caught always in the event of change:
    a young mottled gull stood free on the shoals
    and ate
to vomiting: another gull, squawking possession, cracked a crab,
picked out the entrails, swallowed the soft-shelled legs, a ruddy
turnstone running in to snatch leftover bits:

risk is full: every living thing in
siege: the demand is life, to keep life: the small
white blacklegged egret, how beautiful, quietly stalks and spears
    the shallows, darts to shore
        to stab—what? I couldn't
  see against the black mudflats—a frightened
  fiddler crab?

    the news to my left over the dunes and
reeds and bayberry clumps was
    fall: thousands of tree swallows
    gathering for flight:
    an order held
    in constant change: a congregation
rich with entropy: nevertheless, separable, noticeable
    as one event,

            not chaos: preparations for
flight from winter,
cheet, cheet, cheet, cheet, wings rifling the green clumps,
beaks
at the bayberries
   a perception full of wind, flight, curve,
   sound:
   the possibility of rule as the sum of rulelessness:
the "field" of action
with moving, incalculable center:

in the smaller view, order tight with shape:
blue tiny flowers on a leafless weed: carapace of crab:
snail shell:
        pulsations of order
        in the bellies of minnows: orders swallowed,
broken down, transferred through membranes
to strengthen larger orders: but in the large view, no
lines or changeless shapes: the working in and out, together
        and against, of millions of events: this,
                so that I make
                no form of
                formlessness:

orders as summaries, as outcomes of actions override
or in some way result, not predictably (seeing me gain
the top of a dune,
the swallows
could take flight—some other fields of bayberry
                could enter fall
                berryless) and there is serenity:

                no arranged terror: no forcing of image, plan,
or thought:
no propaganda, no humbling of reality to precept:

terror pervades but is not arranged, all possibilities
of escape open: no route shut, except in
   the sudden loss of all routes:

     I see narrow orders, limited tightness, but will
not run to that easy victory:
     still around the looser, wider forces work:
     I will try
    to fasten into order enlarging grasps of disorder, widening
scope, but enjoying the freedom that
Scope eludes my grasp, that there is no finality of vision,
that I have perceived nothing completely,
    that tomorrow a new walk is a new walk.

John Dyer
THE COUNTRY WALK

The morning's fair; the lusty Sun
With ruddy cheek begins to run;
And early birds, that wing the skies,
Sweetly sing to see him rise.
I am resolv'd, this charming day,
In the open field to stray,
And have no roof above my head,
But that whereon the gods do tread.
Before the yellow barn I see
A beautiful variety
Of strutting cocks, advancing stout,
And flirting empty chaff about:
Hens, ducks, and geese, and all their brood,
And turkeys gobbling for their food,
While rustics thrash the wealthy floor,
And tempt them all to crowd the door.
⠀⠀⠀⠀What a fair face does Nature show!
Augusta! wipe thy dusty brow;
A landscape wide salutes my sight
Of shady vales and mountains bright;
And azure heavens I behold,
And clouds of silver and of gold.
And now into the fields I go,
Where thousand flaming flowers glow,
And every neighb'ring hedge I greet,
With honeysuckle smelling sweet.
Now o'er the daisy-meads I stray,
And meet with, as I pace my way,

Sweetly shining on the eye,
A riv'let gliding smoothly by,
Which shows with what an easy tide
The moments of the happy glide:
Here, finding pleasure after pain,
Sleeping, I see a weary'd swain,
While his full scrip lies open by,
That does his healthy food supply.
Happy swain! sure happier far
Than lofty kings and princes are!
Enjoy sweet sleep, which shuns the crown,
With all its easy beds of down.

     The Sun now shows his noontide blaze,
And sheds around me burning rays.
A little onward, and I go
Into the shade that groves bestow,
And on green moss I lay me down,
That o'er the root of oak has grown;
Where all is silent, but some flood
That sweetly murmurs in the wood;
But birds that warble in the sprays,
And charm ev'n Silence with their lays.

     Oh! pow'rful Silence! How you reign
In the poet's busy brain!
His num'rous thoughts obey the calls
Of the tuneful waterfalls;
Like moles, whene'er the coast is clear,
They rise before thee without fear,
And range in parties here and there.
Some wildly to Parnassus wing,
And view the fair Castalian spring,
Where they behold a lonely well
Where now no tuneful Muses dwell,
But now and then a slavish hind
Paddling the troubled pool they find.

Some trace the pleasing paths of joy,
Others the blissful scene destroy,
In thorny tracks of sorrow stray,
And pine for Clio far away.
But stay—Methinks her lays I hear,
So smooth! so sweet! so deep! so clear!
No, it is not her voice I find;
'Tis but the echo stays behind.

      Some meditate Ambition's brow,
And the black gulph that gapes below;
Some peep in courts, and there they see
The sneaking tribe of Flattery:—
But, striking to the ear and eye,
A nimble deer comes bounding by!
When rushing from yon rustling spray,
It made them vanish all away.
I rouse me up, and on I rove;
'Tis more than time to leave the grove;
The Sun declines, the evening breeze
Begins to whisper through the trees;
And as I leave the sylvan gloom,
As to the glare of day I come,
An old man's smoky nest I see
Leaning on an aged tree,
Whose willow walls, and furzy brow,
A little garden sway below.
Through spreading beds of blooming green,
Matted with herbage sweet and clean,
A vein of water limps along,
And makes them ever green and young.
Here he puffs upon his spade,
And digs up cabbage in the shade;
His tatter'd rags are sable brown,
His beard and hair are hoary grown:
The dying sap descends apace,

And leaves a withered hand and face.
  Up Grongar Hill I labour now,
And catch at last his bushy brow.
Oh! how fresh, how pure the air!
Let me breathe a little here.
Where am I, Nature? I descry
Thy magazine before me lie.
Temples! and towns! and towers! and woods!
And hills! and vales! and fields! and floods!
Crowding before me, edg'd around
With naked wilds, and barren ground.
  See, below, the pleasant dome,
The poet's pride, the poet's home,
Which the sunbeams shine upon,
To the even from the dawn.
See her woods, where Echo talks,
Her gardens trim, her terrace walks,
Her wildernesses, fragrant brakes,
Her gloomy bowers, and shining lakes.
Keep, ye gods! this humble seat
For ever pleasant, private, neat.
  See yonder hill, uprising steep,
Above the river slow and deep;
It looks from hence a pyramid,
Beneath a verdant forest hid;
On whose high top there rises great,
The mighty remnant of a seat,
An old green tow'r, whose batter'd brow
Frowns upon the vale below.
  Look upon that flowery plain,
How the sheep surround their swain,
How they crowd to hear his strain!
All careless with his legs across,
Leaning on a bank of moss,
He spends his empty hours at play,

Which fly as light as down away.
    And there behold a bloomy mead,
A silver stream, a willow shade,
Beneath the shade a fisher stand,
Who, with the angle in his hand,
Swings the nibbling fry to land.
    In blushes the descending sun
Kisses the streams, while slow they run;
And yonder hill remoter grows,
Or dusky clouds do interpose.
The fields are left, the lab'ring hind
His weary oxen does unbind;
And vocal mountains, as they low,
Re-echo to the vales below.
The jocund shepherds piping come,
And drive the herd before them home;
And now begin to light their fires,
Which send up smoke in curling spires;
While with light hearts all homeward tend,
To Aberglasney I descend.
    But oh! how bless'd would be the day,
Did I with Clio pace my way,
And not alone and solitary stray!

Charles Baudelaire
CROWDS

Translated by Roger Gilbert

Taking a bath in a multitude is not for everyone; to enjoy a crowd is an art; and he alone can drink from humanity's vitality upon whom some fairy has in his cradle bestowed a taste for disguises and masks, a hatred of home and a passion for travel.

Multitude, solitude: equal and interchangeable terms for the active and fecund poet. He who does not know how to people his solitude also will not know how to be alone in a busy crowd.

The poet rejoices in this incomparable privilege: that he can in his fashion be both himself and others. Like those wandering souls that search for a body, he can enter whenever he likes into the person of anyone. For him alone, all is vacant; and if certain places appear to be closed to him, it is only because in his eyes they aren't worth the trouble of visiting.

The solitary, pensive walker draws a singular drunkenness from this universal communion. He who can easily blend into the crowd knows feverish pleasures, which will be eternally denied to the egoist, closed like a strong-box, and the sluggard, shut up like a mollusc. He adopts as his own all the professions, all the joys, and all the miseries that circumstances present to him.

That which men call love is quite small, quite restrained and quite weak compared to this ineffable orgy, this holy prostitution of the soul that gives itself entirely, its poetry and its charity, to the unexpected occurrence, the unknown passerby.

It is sometimes good to teach the happy people of the world, if only to humble for an instant their stupid pride, that there are successes superior to theirs, more vast and more refined. The founders of colonies, the shepherds of nations, those missionary priests exiled to the ends of the earth, know something doubtless of these mysterious ecstasies; and, in the bosom of the vast family that their spirit makes for them they must sometimes laugh at those who pity their bad fortunes and their chaste lives.

Frank O'Hara
THE DAY LADY DIED

It is 12:20 in New York a Friday
three days after Bastille day, yes
it is 1959 and I go get a shoeshine
because I will get off the 4:19 in Easthampton
at 7:15 and then go straight to dinner
and I don't know the people who will feed me

I walk up the muggy street beginning to sun
and have a hamburger and a malted and buy
an ugly NEW WORLD WRITING to see what the poets
in Ghana are doing these days
                              I go on to the bank
and Miss Stillwagon (first name Linda I once heard)
doesn't even look up my balance for once in her life
and in the GOLDEN GRIFFIN I get a little Verlaine
for Patsy with drawings by Bonnard although I do
think of Hesiod, trans. Richmond Lattimore or
Brendan Behan's new play or *Le Balcon* or *Les Negres*
of Genet, but I don't, I stick with Verlaine
after practically going to sleep with quandariness

and for Mike I just stroll into the PARK LANE
Liquor Store and ask for a bottle of Strega and
then I go back where I came from to 6th Avenue
and the tobacconist in the Ziegfeld Theatre and
casually ask for a carton of Gauloises and a carton
of Picayunes, and a NEW YORK POST with her face on it

and I am sweating a lot by now and thinking of
leaning on the john door in the 5 SPOT
while she whispered a song along the keyboard
to Mal Waldron and everyone and I stopped breathing

James Joyce
AN ENCOUNTER

It was Joe Dillon who introduced the Wild West to us. He had a little library made up of old numbers of *The Union Jack, Pluck,* and *The Halfpenny Marvel.* Every evening after school we met in his back garden and arranged Indian battles. He and his fat young brother Leo, the idler, held the loft of the stable while we tried to carry it by storm; or we fought a pitched battle on the grass. But, however well we fought, we never won siege or battle and all our bouts ended with Joe Dillon's war dance of victory. His parents went to eight o'clock mass every morning in Gardiner Street and the peaceful odour of Mrs Dillon was prevalent in the hall of the house. But he played too fiercely for us who were younger and more timid. He looked like some kind of an Indian when he capered round the garden, an old tea-cosy on his head, beating a tin with his fist and yelling:

'Ya! yaka, yaka, yaka!'

Everyone was incredulous when it was reported that he had a vocation for the priesthood. Nevertheless it was true.

A spirit of unruliness diffused itself among us and, under its influence, differences of culture and constitution were waived. We banded ourselves together, some boldly, some in jest and some almost in fear: and of the number of these latter, the reluctant Indians who were afraid to seem studious or lacking in robustness, I was one. The adventures related in the literature of the Wild West were remote from my nature but, at least, they opened doors of escape. I liked better some American detective stories which were traversed from time to time by unkempt fierce and beautiful girls. Though there was nothing wrong in these stories and though their intention was sometimes literary they were circulated secretly at school. One day when Father Butler was hearing the four pages of Roman History clumsy Leo Dillon was discovered with a copy of *The Halfpenny Marvel.*

'This page or this page? This page? Now, Dillon, up!" Hardly had the day"... Go on! What day? "Hardly had the day dawned"... Have you studied it? What have you there in your pocket?'

Everyone's heart palpitated as Leo Dillon handed up the paper and everyone assumed an innocent face. Father Butler turned over the pages, frowning.

'What is this rubbish?' he said. '*The Apache Chief!* Is this what you read instead of studying your Roman History? Let me not find any more of this wretched stuff in this college. The man who wrote it, I suppose, was some wretched scribbler that writes these things for a drink. I'm surprised at boys like you, educated, reading such stuff. I could understand it if you were ... National School boys. Now, Dillon, I advise you strongly, get at your work or ... '

This rebuke during the sober hours of school paled much of the glory of the Wild West for me, and the confused puffy face of Leo Dillon awakened one of my consciences. But when the restraining influence of the school was at a distance I began to hunger again for wild sensations, for the escape which those chronicles of disorder alone seemed to offer me. The mimic warfare of the evening became at last as wearisome to me as the routine of school in the morning because I wanted real adventures to happen to myself. But real adventures, I reflected, do not happen to people who remain at home: they must be sought abroad.

The summer holidays were near at hand when I made up my mind to break out of the weariness of school-life for one day at least. With Leo Dillon and a boy named Mahony I planned a day's miching. Each of us saved up sixpence. We were to meet at ten in the morning on the Canal Bridge. Mahony's big sister was to write an excuse for him and Leo Dillon was to tell his brother to say he was sick. We arranged to go along the Wharf Road until we came to the ships, then to cross in the ferryboat and walk out to see the Pigeon House. Leo Dillon was afraid we might meet Father Butler or someone out of the college; but Mahony asked, very sensibly, what would Father Butler be doing out at the Pigeon House. We were reassured: and I brought the first stage of the plot to an end by collecting sixpence from the other two, at the same time showing them my own sixpence. When we were making the last arrangements on the eve we were all vaguely excited. We shook hands, laughing, and Mahony said:

'Till tomorrow, mates.'

That night I slept badly. In the morning I was firstcomer to the bridge as I lived nearest. I hid my books in the long grass near the ashpit at the end of the garden where nobody ever came and hurried along the canal bank. It was a mild sunny morning in the first week of June. I sat up on the coping of the bridge admiring my frail canvas shoes which I had diligently pipeclayed overnight and watching the docile horses pulling a tramload of business people up the hill. All the branches of the tall trees which lined the mall were gay with little light green leaves and the sunlight slanted through them on to the water. The granite stone of the bridge was beginning to be warm and I began to pat it with my hands in time to an air in my head. I was very happy.

When I had been sitting there for five or ten minutes I saw Mahony's grey suit approaching. He came up the hill, smiling, and clambered up beside me on the bridge. While we were waiting he brought out the catapult which bulged from his inner pocket and explained some improvements which he had made in it. I asked him why he had brought it and he told me he had brought it to have some gas with the birds. Mahony used slang freely, and spoke of Father Butler as Bunser Burner. We waited on for a quarter of an hour more, but still there was no sign of Leo Dillon. Mahony, at last, jumped down and said:

'Come along. I knew Fatty'd funk it.'

'And his sixpence . . . ?' I said.

'That's forfeit,' said Mahony. 'And so much the better for us—a bob and a tanner instead of a bob.'

We walked along the North Strand Road till we came to the Vitriol Works and then turned to the right along the Wharf Road. Mahony began to play the Indian as soon as we were out of public sight. He chased a crowd of ragged girls, brandishing his unloaded catapult and, when two ragged boys began, out of chivalry, to fling stones at us, he proposed that we should charge them. I objected that the boys were too small, and so we walked on, the ragged troop screaming after us 'Swaddlers! Swaddlers!' thinking that we were Protestants because Mahony, who was dark-complexioned, wore the silver badge of a cricket club in his cap. When we came to the Smoothing Iron we arranged a siege; but it was a failure because you must have at least three. We revenged ourselves on Leo Dillon by saying what a funk he was and guessing how many he would get at three o'clock from Mr Ryan.

We came then near the river. We spent a long time walking about the noisy streets flanked by high stone walls, watching the working of cranes and engines and often being shouted at for our immobility by the drivers of groaning carts. It was noon when we reached the quays and, as all the labourers seemed to be eating their lunches, we bought two big currant buns and sat down to eat them on some metal piping beside the river. We pleased ourselves with the spectacle of Dublin's commerce—the barges signalled from far away by their curls of woolly smoke, the brown fishing fleet beyond Ringsend, the big white sailing-vessel which was being discharged on the opposite quay. Mahony said it would be right skit to run away to sea on one of those big ships, and even I, looking at the high masts, saw, or imagined, the geography which had been scantily dosed to me at school gradually taking substance under my eyes. School and home seemed to recede from us and their influences upon us seemed to wane.

We crossed the Liffey in the ferryboat, paying our toll to be transported in the company of two labourers and a little Jew with a bag. We were serious to the point of solemnity, but once during the short voyage our eyes met and we laughed. When we landed we watched the discharging of the graceful three-master which we had observed from the other quay. Some bystander said that she was a Norwegian vessel. I went to the stern and tried to decipher the legend upon it but, failing to do so, I came back and examined the foreign sailors to see had any of them green eyes for I had some confused notion. . . . The sailors' eyes were blue and grey and even black. The only sailor whose eyes could have been called green was a tall man who amused the crowd on the quay by calling out cheerfully every time the planks fell:

'All right! All right!'

When we were tired of this sight we wandered slowly into Ringsend. The day had grown sultry, and in the windows of the grocers' shops musty biscuits lay bleaching. We bought some biscuits and chocolate which we ate sedulously as we wandered through the squalid streets where the families of the fishermen live. We could find no dairy and so we went into a huckster's shop and bought a bottle of raspberry lemonade each. Refreshed by this, Mahony chased a cat down a lane, but the cat escaped into a wide field. We both felt rather tired and when we reached the field we made at once for a sloping bank over the ridge of which we could see the Dodder.

It was too late and we were too tired to carry out our project of visiting the

Pigeon House. We had to be home before four o'clock lest our adventure should be discovered. Mahony looked regretfully at his catapult and I had to suggest going home by train before he regained any cheerfulness. The sun went in behind some clouds and left us to our jaded thoughts and the crumbs of our provisions.

There was nobody but ourselves in the field. When we had lain on the bank for some time without speaking I saw a man approaching from the far end of the field. I watched him lazily as I chewed one of those green stems on which girls tell fortunes. He came along by the bank slowly. He walked with one hand upon his hip and in the other hand he held a stick with which he tapped the turf lightly. He was shabbily dressed in a suit of greenish-black and wore what we used to call a jerry hat with a high crown. He seemed to be fairly old for his moustache was ashen-grey. When he passed at our feet he glanced up at us quickly and then continued his way. We followed him with our eyes and saw that when he had gone on for perhaps fifty paces he turned about and began to retrace his steps. He walked towards us very slowly, always tapping the ground with his stick, so slowly that I thought he was looking for something in the grass.

He stopped when he came level with us and bade us good-day. We answered him and he sat down beside us on the slope slowly and with great care. He began to talk of the weather, saying that it would be a very hot summer and adding that the seasons had changed greatly since he was a boy—a long time ago. He said that the happiest time of one's life was undoubtedly one's schoolboy days and that he would give anything to be young again. While he expressed these sentiments which bored us a little, we kept silent. Then he began to talk of school and of books. He asked us whether we had read the poetry of Thomas Moore or the works of Sir Walter Scott and Lord Lytton. I pretended that I had read every book he mentioned so that in the end he said:

'Ah, I can see you are a bookworm like myself. Now,' he added, pointing to Mahony, who was regarding us with open eyes, 'he is different; he goes in for games.'

He said he had all Sir Walter Scott's works and all Lord Lytton's works at home and never tired of reading them. 'Of course,' he said, 'there were some of Lord Lytton's works which boys couldn't read.' Mahony asked why couldn't boys read them—a question which agitated and pained me because I was afraid the man would think I was as stupid as Mahony. The man, however, only smiled. I saw that he had great gaps in his mouth between his yellow teeth. Then he asked us which of us had the most sweethearts. Mahony mentioned lightly that he had three totties. The man asked me how many had I. I answered that I had none. He did not believe me and said he was sure I must have one. I was silent.

'Tell us,' said Mahony pertly to the man, 'how many have you yourself?'

The man smiled as before and said that when he was our age he had lots of sweethearts.

'Every boy,' he said, 'has a little sweetheart.'

His attitude on this point struck me as strangely liberal in a man of his age. In my heart I thought that what he said about boys and sweethearts was reasonable. But I disliked the words in his mouth and I wondered why he shivered once or twice as if he feared something or felt a sudden chill. As he proceeded I noticed that his accent was good. He began to speak to us about girls, saying what nice soft hair they had and how soft their hands were and how all girls were not so good as they seemed to be if one only knew. There was nothing he liked, he said, so much as looking at a nice young girl, at her nice white hands and her beautiful soft hair. He gave me the impression that he was repeating something which he had learned by heart or that, magnetised by some words of his own speech, his mind was slowly circling round and round in the same orbit. At times he spoke as if he were simply alluding to some fact that everybody knew, and at times he lowered his voice and spoke mysteriously, as if he were telling us something secret which he did not wish others to overhear. He repeated his phrases over and over again, varying them and surrounding them with his monotonous voice. I continued to gaze towards the foot of the slope, listening to him.

After a long while his monologue paused. He stood up slowly, saying that he had to leave us for a minute or so, a few minutes, and, without changing the direction of my gaze, I saw him walking slowly away from us towards the near end of the field. We remained silent when he had gone. After a silence of a few minutes I heard Mahony exclaim:

'I say! Look what he's doing!'

As I neither answered nor raised my eyes, Mahony exclaimed again:

'I say . . . He's a queer old josser!'

'In case he asks us for our names,' I said, 'let you be Murphy and I'll be Smith.'

We said nothing further to each other. I was still considering whether I would go away or not when the man came back and sat down beside us again. Hardly had he sat down when Mahony, catching sight of the cat which had escaped him, sprang up and pursued her across the field. The man and I watched the chase. The cat escaped once more and Mahony began to throw stones at the wall she had escaladed. Desisting from this, he began to wander about the far end of the field, aimlessly.

After an interval the man spoke to me. He said that my friend was a very rough boy, and asked did he get whipped often at school. I was going to reply indignantly that we were not National School boys to be *whipped*, as he called it; but I remained silent. He began to speak on the subject of chastising boys. His mind, as if magnetised again by his speech, seemed to circle slowly round and round its new centre. He said that when boys were that kind they ought to be whipped and well whipped. When a boy was rough and unruly there was nothing would do him any good but a good sound whipping. A slap on the hand or a box on the ear was no good: what he wanted was to get a nice warm whipping. I was surprised at this sentiment and involuntarily glanced at his face. As I did so I met the gaze of a pair of bottle-green eyes peering at me from under a twitching forehead. I turned my eyes away again.

The man continued his monologue. He seemed to have forgotten his recent liberalism. He said that if ever he found a boy talking to girls or having a girl for a sweetheart he would whip him and whip him; and that would teach him not to be talking to girls. And if a boy had a girl for a sweetheart and told lies about it, then he would give him such a whipping as no boy ever got in this world. He said that there was nothing in this world he would like so well as that. He described to me how he would whip such a boy as if he were unfolding some elaborate mystery. He would love that, he said, better than anything in this world; and his voice, as he led me monotonously through the mystery, grew almost affectionate and seemed to plead with me that I should understand him.

I waited till his monologue paused again. Then I stood up abruptly. Lest I should betray my agitation I delayed a few moments pretending to fix my shoe properly and then, saying that I was obliged to go, I bade him good-day. I went up the slope calmly but my heart was beating quickly with fear that he would seize me by the ankles. When I reached the top of the slope I turned round and, without looking at him, called loudly across the field:

'Murphy!'

My voice had an accent of forced bravery in it, and I was ashamed of my paltry stratagem. I had to call the name again before Mahony saw me and hallooed in answer. How my heart beat as he came running across the field to me! He ran as if to bring me aid. And I was penitent; for in my heart I had always despised him a little.

Elizabeth Bishop
THE END OF MARCH

For John Malcolm Brinnin and Bill Read: Duxbury

It was cold and windy, scarcely the day
to take a walk on that long beach.
Everything was withdrawn as far as possible,
indrawn: the tide far out, the ocean shrunken,
seabirds in ones or twos.
The rackety, icy, offshore wind
numbed our faces on one side;
disrupted the formation
of a lone flight of Canada geese;
and blew back the low, inaudible rollers
in upright, steely mist.

The sky was darker than the water
—*it* was the color of mutton-fat jade.
Along the wet sand, in rubber boots, we followed
a track of big dog-prints (so big
they were more like lion-prints). Then we came on
lengths and lengths, endless, of wet white string,
looping up to the tide-line, down to the water,
over and over. Finally, they did end:
a thick white snarl, man-size, awash,
rising on every wave, a sodden ghost,
falling back, sodden, giving up the ghost. . . .
A kite string?—But no kite.

I wanted to get as far as my proto-dream-house,
my crypto-dream-house, that crooked box
set up on pilings, shingled green,
a sort of artichoke of a house, but greener
(boiled with bicarbonate of soda?),
protected from spring tides by a palisade
of—are they railroad ties?
(Many things about this place are dubious.)
I'd like to retire there and do *nothing,*
or nothing much, forever, in two bare rooms:
look through binoculars, read boring books,
old, long, long books, and write down useless notes,
talk to myself, and, foggy days,
watch the droplets slipping, heavy with light.
At night, a *grog à l'américaine.*
I'd blaze it with a kitchen match
and lovely, diaphanous blue flame
would waver, doubled in the window.
There must be a stove; there *is* a chimney,
askew, but braced with wires,
and electricity, possibly
—at least, at the back another wire
limply leashes the whole affair
to something off behind the dunes.
A light to read by—perfect! But—impossible.
And that day the wind was much too cold
even to get that far,
and of course the house was boarded up.

On the way back our faces froze on the other side.
The sun came out for just a minute.
For just a minute, set in their bezels of sand,
the drab, damp, scattered stones
were multi-colored,
and all those high enough threw out long shadows,

individual shadows, then pulled them in again.
They could have been teasing the lion sun,
except that now he was behind them
—a sun who'd walked the beach the last low tide,
making those big, majestic paw-prints,
who perhaps had batted a kite out of the sky to play with.

Alice Meynell
THE FOOT

Time was when no good news made a journey, and no friend came near, but a welcome was uttered, or at least thought, for the travelling feet of the wayfarer or the herald. The feet, the feet were beautiful on the mountains; their toil was the price of all communication, and their reward the first service and refreshment. They were blessed and bathed; they suffered, but they were friends with the earth; dews in grass at morning, shallow rivers at noon, gave them coolness. They must have grown hard upon their mountain paths, yet never so hard but they needed and had the first pity and the readiest succour. It was never easy for the feet of man to travel this earth, shod or unshod, and his feet are delicate, like his colour.

If they suffered hardship once, they suffer privation now. Yet the feet should have more of the acquaintance of earth, and know more of flowers, freshness, cool brooks, wild thyme, and salt sand than does anything else about us. It is their calling; and the hands might be glad to be stroked for a day by grass and struck by buttercups, as the feet are of those who go barefoot; and the nostrils might be flattered to be, like them, so long near moss. The face has only now and then, for a resting-while, their privilege.

If our feet are now so severed from the natural ground, they have inevitably lost life and strength by the separation. It is only the entirely unshod that have lively feet. Watch a peasant who never wears shoes, except for a few unkind hours once a week, and you may see the play of his talk in his mobile feet; they become as dramatic as his hands. Fresh as the air, brown with the light, and healthy from the field, not used to darkness, not grown in prison, the foot of the *contadino* is not abashed. It is the foot of high life that is prim, and never lifts a heel against its dull conditions, for it has forgotten liberty. It is more active now than it lately was—certainly the foot of woman is more active; but whether on the pedal or in the stirrup, or clad for a walk, or armed for a game, or decked for the waltz, it is in bonds. It is, at any rate, inarticulate.

It has no longer a distinct and divided life, or none that is visible and sensible. Whereas the whole living body has naturally such infinite distinctness that the sense of touch differs, as it were, with every nerve, and the fingers are so separate that it was believed of them of old that each one had its angel, yet the modern foot is, as much as possible, deprived of all that delicate distinction: undone, unspecialized, sent back to lower forms of indiscriminate life. It is as though a landscape with separate sweetness in every tree should be rudely painted with the blank—blank, not simple—generalities of a vulgar hand. Or as though one should take the pleasures of a day of happiness in a wholesale fashion, not "turning the hours to moments," which joy can do to the full as perfectly as pain.

The foot, with its articulations, is suppressed, and its language confused. When Lovelace likens the hand of Amarantha to a violin, and her glove to the case, he has at any rate a glove to deal with, not a boot. Yet Amarantha's foot is as lovely as her hand. It, too, has a "tender inward"; no wayfaring would ever make it look anything but delicate; its arch seems too slight to carry her through a night of dances; it does, in fact, but balance her. It is fit to cling to the ground, but rather for springing than for rest.

And, doubtless, for man, woman, and child the tender, irregular, sensitive, living foot, which does not even stand with all its little surface on the ground, and which makes no base to satisfy an architectural eye, is, as it were, the unexpected thing. It is a part of vital design and has a history; and man does not go erect but at a price of weariness and pain. How weak it is may be seen from a footprint: for nothing makes a more helpless and unsymmetrical sign than does a naked foot.

Tender, too, is the silence of human feet. You have but to pass a season amongst the barefooted to find that man, who, shod, makes so much ado, is naturally as silent as snow. Woman, who not only makes her armed heel heard, but also goes rustling like a shower, is naturally silent as snow. The vintager is not heard among the vines, nor the harvester on his threshing-floor of stone. There is a kind of simple stealth in their coming and going, and they show sudden smiles and dark eyes in and out of the rows of harvest when you thought yourself alone. The lack of noise in their movement sets free the sound of their voices, and their laughter floats.

But we shall not praise the "simple, sweet" and "earth-confiding feet" enough without thanks for the rule of verse and for the time of song. If Poetry was first divided by the march, and next varied by the dance, then to the rule of the foot are to be ascribed the thought, the instruction, and the dream that could not speak by prose. Out of that little physical law, then, grew a spiritual law which is one of the greatest things we know; and from the test of the foot came the ultimate test of the thinker: "Is it accepted of Song?"

The monastery, in like manner, holds its sons to little trivial rules of time and exactitude, not to be broken, laws that are made secure against the restlessness of the heart fretting for insignificant liberties—trivial laws to restrain from a trivial freedom. And within the gate of these laws which seem so small, lies the world of mystic virtue. They enclose, they imply, they lock, they answer for it. Lesser virtues may flower in daily liberty and may flourish in prose; but infinite virtues and greatness are compelled to the measure of poetry, and obey the constraint of an hourly convent bell. It is no wonder that every poet worthy the name has had a passion for metre, for the very verse. To him the difficult fetter is the condition of an interior range immeasurable.

Nathaniel Hawthorne
FOOT-PRINTS ON THE SEA-SHORE

It must be a spirit much unlike my own, which can keep itself in health and vigor without sometimes stealing from the sultry sunshine of the world, to plunge into the cool bath of solitude. At intervals, and not infrequent ones, the forest and the ocean summon me—one with the roar of its waves, the other with the murmur of its boughs—forth from the haunts of men. But I must wander many a mile, ere I could stand beneath the shadow of even one primeval tree, much less be lost among the multitude of hoary trunks, and hidden from earth and sky by the mystery of darksome foliage. Nothing is within my daily reach more like a forest than the acre or two of woodland near some suburban farmhouse. When, therefore, the yearning for seclusion becomes a necessity within me, I am drawn to the sea-shore, which extends its line of rude rocks and seldom-trodden sands, for leagues around our bay. Setting forth, at my last ramble, on a September morning, I bound myself with a hermit's vow, to interchange no thoughts with man or woman, to share no social pleasure, but to derive all that day's enjoyment from shore, and sea, and sky,—from my soul's communion with these, and from fantasies, and recollections, or anticipated realities. Surely here is enough to feed a human spirit for a single day. Farewell, then, busy world! 'Till your evening lights shall shine along the street—'till they gleam upon my sea-flushed face, as I tread homeward—free me from your ties, and let me be a peaceful outlaw.

Highways and cross-paths are hastily traversed; and, clambering down a crag, I find myself at the extremity of a long beach. How gladly does the spirit leap forth, and suddenly enlarge its sense of being to the full extent of the broad, blue, sunny deep! A greeting and a homage to the Sea! I descend over its margin, and dip my hand into the wave that meets me, and bathe my brow. That far-resounding roar is Ocean's voice of welcome. His salt breath brings a blessing along with it. Now let us pace together—the reader's fancy arm in arm with mine—this noble beach, which extends a mile or more from that craggy promontory to yonder rampart of broken rocks. In front, the sea; in the rear, a precipitous bank, the grassy verge of which is breaking away, year after year, and flings down its tufts of verdure upon the barrenness below. The beach itself is a broad space of sand, brown and sparkling, with hardly any pebbles intermixed. Near the water's edge there is a wet margin, which glistens brightly in the sunshine, and reflects objects like a mirror; and as we tread along the glistening border, a dry spot flashes around each footstep, but grows moist again, as we lift our feet. In some spots, the sand receives a complete impression of the sole—square toe and all; elsewhere, it is of such marble firmness, that we must stamp heavily to leave a print even of the iron-shod heel. Along the whole of this extensive beach gambols the surf-wave; now it makes a feint of dashing onward in a fury, yet dies away with a meek murmur, and does but kiss the strand; now, after many such abortive efforts, it rears itself up in an unbroken line, heightening as it advances, without a speck of foam on its green crest. With how fierce a roar it flings itself forward, and rushes far up the beach!

As I threw my eyes along the edge of the surf, I remember that I was startled, as Robinson Crusoe might have been, by the sense that human life was within the magic circle of my solitude. Afar off in the remote distance of the beach, appearing like sea-nymphs, or some airier things, such as might tread upon the feathery spray, was a group of girls. Hardly had I beheld them, when they passed into the shadow of the rocks and vanished. To comfort myself— for truly I would fain have gazed a while longer—I made acquaintance with a flock of beach-birds. These little citizens of the sea and air preceded me by about a stone's-throw along the strand, seeking, I suppose, for food upon its margin. Yet, with a philosophy which mankind would do well to imitate, they drew a continual pleasure from their toil for a subsistence. The sea was each little bird's great playmate. They chased it downward as it swept back, and again ran up swiftly before the impending wave, which sometimes overtook them and bore them off their feet. But they floated as lightly as one of their own feathers on the breaking crest. In their airy flutterings, they seemed to rest on the evanescent spray. Their images,—long-legged little figures, with grey backs and snowy bosoms,—were seen as distinctly as the realities in the mirror of the glistening strand. As I advanced, they flew a score or two of yards, and, again alighting, recommenced their dalliance with the surf-wave; and thus they bore me company along the beach, the types of pleasant fantasies, 'till, at its extremity, they took wing over the ocean, and were gone. After forming a friendship with these small surf-spirits, it is really worth a sigh, to find no memorial of them save their multitudinous little tracks in the sand.

When we have paced the length of the beach, it is pleasant, and not unprofitable, to retrace our steps, and recall the whole mood and occupation of the mind during the former passage. Our tracks, being all discernible, will guide us with an observing consciousness through every unconscious wandering of thought and fancy. Here we followed the surf in its reflux, to pick up a shell which the sea seemed loath to relinquish. Here we found a sea-weed, with an immense brown leaf, and trailed it behind us by its long snake-like stalk. Here we seized a live horse-shoe by the tail, and counted the many claws of that queer monster. Here we dug into the sand for pebbles, and skipped them upon the surface of the water. Here we wet our feet while examining a jelly-fish, which the waves, having just tossed it up, now sought to snatch away again. Here we trod along the brink of a fresh-water brooklet, which flows across the beach, becoming shallower and more shallow, 'till at last it sinks into the sand, and perishes in the effort to bear its little tribute to the main. Here some vagary appears to have bewildered us; for our tracks go round and round, and are confusedly intermingled, as if we had found a labyrinth upon the level beach. And here, amid our idle pastime, we sat down upon almost the only stone that breaks the surface of the sand, and were lost in an unlooked-for and overpowering conception of the majesty and awfulness of the great deep. Thus, by tracking our foot-prints in the sand, we track our own nature in its wayward course, and steal a glance upon it, when it never dreams of being so observed. Such glances always make us wiser.

This extensive beach affords room for another pleasant pastime. With your staff, you may write verses—love-verses, if they please you best—and consecrate them with a woman's name. Here, too, may be inscribed thoughts, feelings, desires, warm outgushings from the heart's secret places, which one would not pour upon the sand without the certainty that, almost ere the sky has looked upon them, the sea will wash them out. Stir not hence, 'till the record be effaced. Now—for there is room enough on your canvass—draw huge faces—huge as that of the Sphynx on Egyptian sands—and fit them with bodies of corresponding immensity, and legs which might stride half-way to yonder island. Child's play becomes magnificent on so grand a scale. But, after all, the most fascinating employment is simply to write your name in the sand. Draw the letters gigantic, so that two strides may barely measure them, and three for the long strokes! Cut deep, that the record may be permanent! Statesmen, and warriors, and poets, have spent their strength in no better cause than this. Is it accomplished? Return, then, in an hour or two, and seek for this mighty record of a name. The sea will have swept over it, even as time rolls its effacing waves over the names of statesmen, and warriors, and poets. Hark, the surf-wave laughs at you!

Passing from the beach, I begin to clamber over the crags, making my difficult way among the ruins of a rampart, shattered and broken by the assaults of a fierce enemy. The rocks rise in every variety of attitude; some of them have their feet in the foam, and are shagged half-way upward with sea-weed; some have been hollowed almost into caverns by the unwearied toil of the sea, which can afford to spend centuries in wearing away a rock, or even polishing a pebble. One huge rock ascends in monumental shape, with a face like a giant's tombstone, on which the veins resemble inscriptions, but in an unknown tongue. We will fancy them the forgotten characters of an antediluvian race; or else that nature's own hand has here recorded a mystery, which, could I read her language, would make mankind the wiser and the happier. How many a thing has troubled me with that same idea! Pass on, and leave it unexplained. Here is a narrow avenue, which might seem to have been hewn through the very heart of an enormous crag, affording passage for the rising sea to thunder back and forth, filling it with tumultuous foam, and then leaving its floor of black pebbles bare and glistening. In this chasm there was once an intersecting vein of softer stone, which the waves have gnawed away piecemeal, while the granite walls remain entire on either side. How sharply, and with what harsh clamor, does the sea rake back the pebbles, as it momentarily withdraws into its own depths! At intervals, the floor of the chasm is left nearly dry; but anon, at the outlet, two or three great waves are seen struggling to get in at once; two hit the walls athwart, which one rushes straight through, and all three thunder, as if with rage and triumph. They heap the chasm with a snow-drift of foam and spray. While watching this scene, I can never rid myself of the idea, that a monster, endowed with life and fierce energy, is striving to burst his way through the narrow pass. And what a contrast, to look through the stormy chasm, and catch a glimpse of the calm bright sea beyond!

Many interesting discoveries may be made along these broken cliffs. Once, for example, I found a dead seal, which a recent tempest had tossed into a nook of the rocks, where his shaggy carcass lay rolled in a heap of eel-grass, as if the sea-monster sought to hide himself from my eye. Another time, a shark seemed on the point of leaping from the surf to swallow me; nor did I, wholly without dread, approach near enough to ascertain that the man-eater had already met his own death from some fisherman in the bay. In the same ramble, I encountered a bird—a large grey bird—but whether a loon, or a wild goose, or the identical albatross of the Ancient Mariner, was beyond my ornithology to decide. It reposed so naturally on a bed of dry sea-weed, with its head beside its wing, that I almost fancied it alive, and trod softly lest it should suddenly spread its wings skyward. But the sea-bird would soar among the clouds no more, nor ride upon its native waves; so I drew near, and pulled out one of its mottled tail-feathers for a remembrance. Another day, I discovered an immense bone, wedged into a chasm of the rocks; it was at least ten feet long, curved like a scimitar, bejewelled with barnacles and small shell-fish, and partly covered with a growth of sea-weed. Some leviathan of former ages had used this ponderous mass as a jaw-bone. Curiosities of a minuter order may be observed in a deep reservoir, which is replenished with water at every tide, but becomes a lake among the crags, save when the sea is at its height. At the bottom of this rocky basin grow marine plants, some of which tower high beneath the water, and cast a shadow in the sunshine. Small fishes dart to and fro, and hide themselves among the sea-weed; there is also a solitary crab, who appears to lead the life of a hermit, communing with none of the other denizens of the place; and likewise several five-fingers—for I know no other name than that which children give them. If your imagination be at all accustomed to such freaks, you may look down into the depths of this pool, and fancy it the mysterious depth of ocean. But where are the hulks and scattered timbers of sunken ships?—where the treasures that old Ocean hoards?—where the corroded cannon?—where the corpses and skeletons of seamen, who went down in storm and battle?

On the day of my last ramble, (it was a September day, yet as warm as summer,) what should I behold as I approached the above described basin but three girls sitting on its margin, and—yes, it is veritably so—laving their snowy feet in the sunny water! These, these are the warm realities of those three visionary shapes that flitted from me on the beach. Hark! their merry voices, as they toss up the water with their feet! They have not seen me. I must shrink behind this rock, and steal away again.

In honest truth, vowed to solitude as I am, there is something in the encounter that makes the heart flutter with a strangely pleasant sensation. I know these girls to be realities of flesh and blood, yet, glancing at them so briefly, they mingle like kindred creatures with the ideal beings of my mind. It is pleasant, likewise, to gaze down from some high crag, and watch a group of children, gathering pebbles and pearly shells, and playing with the surf, as with old Ocean's hoary beard. Nor does it infringe upon my seclusion, to see yonder boat at anchor off the shore, swinging dreamily to and fro, and rising and sinking with the alternate swell; while the crew—four gentlemen in round-about jackets—are busy with their fishing-lines. But, with an inward antipathy and a headlong flight, do I eschew the presence of any meditative stroller like myself, known by his pilgrim staff, his sauntering step, his shy demeanor, his observant yet abstracted eye. From such a man, as if another self had scared me, I scramble hastily over the rocks and take refuge in a nook which many a secret hour has given me a right to call my own. I would do battle for it even with the churl that should produce the title-deeds. Have not my musings melted into its rocky walls and sandy floor, and made them a portion of myself?

It is a recess in the line of cliffs, walled round by a rough, high precipice, which almost encircles and shuts in a little space of sand. In front, the sea appears as between the pillars of a portal. In the rear, the precipice is broken and intermixed with earth, which gives nourishment not only to clinging and twining shrubs, but to trees, that grip the rock with their naked roots, and seem to struggle hard for footing and for soil enough to live upon. These are fir trees; but oaks hang their heavy branches from above, and throw down acorns on the beach, and shed their withering foliage upon the waves. At this autumnal season, the precipice is decked with variegated splendor; trailing wreaths of scarlet flaunt from the summit downward; tufts of yellow-flowering shrubs, and rose bushes, with their reddened leaves and glossy seed-berries, sprout from each crevice; at every glance, I detect some new light or shade of beauty, all contrasting with the stern, grey rock. A rill of water trickles down the cliff and fills a little cistern near the base. I drain it at a draught, and find it fresh and pure. This recess shall be my dining-hall. And what the feast? A few biscuits, made savory by soaking them in sea-water, a tuft of samphire gathered from the beach, and an apple for the dessert. By this time, the little rill has filled its reservoir again; and, as I quaff it, I thank God more heartily than for a civic banquet, that He gives me the healthful appetite to make a feast of bread and water.

Dinner being over, I throw myself at length upon the sand, and basking in the sunshine, let my mind disport itself at will. The walls of this my hermitage have no tongue to tell my follies, though I sometimes fancy that they have ears to hear them, and a soul to sympathize. There is a magic in this spot. Dreams haunt its precincts, and flit around me in broad sunlight, nor require that sleep shall blindfold me to real objects, ere these be visible. Here can I frame a story of two lovers, and make their shadows live before me, and be mirrored in the tranquil water, as they tread along the sand, leaving no foot-prints. Here, should I will it, I can summon up a single shade, and be myself her lover. Yes, dreamer,—but your lonely heart will be the colder for such fancies. Sometimes, too, the Past comes back, and finds me here, and in her train come faces which were gladsome, when I knew them, yet seem not gladsome now. Would that my hiding place were lonelier, so that the Past might not find me! Get ye all gone, old friends, and let me listen to the murmur of the sea,—a melancholy voice, but less sad than yours. Of what mysteries is it telling? Of sunken ships, and whereabouts they lie? Of islands afar and undiscovered, whose tawny children are unconscious of other islands and of continents, and deem the stars of heaven their nearest neighbours? Nothing of all this. What then? Has it talked for so many ages, and meant nothing all the while? No; for those ages find utterance in the sea's unchanging voice, and warn the listener to withdraw his interest from mortal vicissitudes, and let the infinite idea of eternity pervade his soul. This is wisdom; and, therefore, will I spend the next half-hour in shaping little boats of drift-wood, and launching them on voyages across the cove, with the feather of a sea-gull for a sail. If the voice of ages tell me true, this is as wise an occupation as to build ships of five hundred tons, and launch them forth upon the main, bound to "far Cathay." Yet, how would the merchant sneer at me!

And, after all, can such philosophy be true? Methinks I could find a thousand arguments against it. Well, then, let yonder shaggy rock, mid-deep in the surf—see! he is somewhat wrathful,—he rages and roars and foams—let that tall rock be my antagonist, and let me exercise my oratory like him of Athens, who bandied words with an angry sea and got the victory. My maiden speech is a triumphant one; for the gentleman in sea-weed has nothing to offer in reply, save an immitigable roaring. His voice, indeed, will be heard a long while after mine is hushed. Once more I shout, and the cliffs reverberate the sound. Oh, what joy for a shy man to feel himself so solitary, that he may lift his voice to its highest pitch without hazard of a listener! But, hush!—be silent, my good friend!—whence comes that stifled laughter? It was musical,—but how should there be such music in my solitude? Looking upwards, I catch a glimpse of three faces, peeping from the summit of the cliff, like angels between me and their native sky. Ah, fair girls, you may make yourselves merry at my eloquence,—but it was my turn to smile when I saw your white feet in the pool! Let us keep each other's secrets.

The sunshine has now passed from my hermitage, except a gleam upon the sand just where it meets the sea. A crowd of gloomy fantasies will come and haunt me, if I tarry longer here, in the darkening twilight of these grey rocks. This is a dismal place in some moods of the mind. Climb we, therefore, the precipice, and pause a moment on the brink, gazing down into that hollow chamber by the deep, where we have been, what few can be, sufficient to our own pastime—yes, say the word outright!—self-sufficient to our own happiness. How lonesome looks the recess now, and dreary too,—like all other spots where happiness has been! There lies my shadow in the departing sunshine with its head upon the sea. I will pelt it with pebbles. A hit! a hit! I clap my hands in triumph, and see my shadow clapping its unreal hands, and claiming the triumph for itself. What a simpleton must I have been all day, since my own shadow makes a mock of my fooleries!

Homeward! homeward! It is time to hasten home. It is time; it is time; for as the sun sinks over the western wave, the sea grows melancholy, and the surf has a saddened tone. The distant sails appear astray, and not of earth, in their remoteness amid the desolate waste. My spirit wanders forth afar, but finds no resting place, and comes shivering back. It is time that I were hence. But grudge me not the day that has been spent in seclusion, which yet was not solitude, since the great sea has been my companion, and the little sea-birds my friends, and the wind has told me his secrets, and airy shapes have flitted around me in my hermitage. Such companionship works an effect upon a man's character, as if he had been admitted to the society of creatures that are not mortal. And when, at noontide, I tread the crowded streets, the influence of this day will still be felt; so that I shall walk among men kindly and as a brother, with affection and sympathy, but yet shall not melt into the indistinguishable mass of humankind. I shall think my own thoughts, and feel my own emotions, and possess my individuality unviolated.

But it is good, at the eve of such a day, to feel and know that there are men and women in the world. That feeling and that knowledge are mine, at this moment; for, on the shore, far below me, the fishing-party have landed from their skiff, and are cooking their scaly prey by a fire of drift-wood, kindled in the angle of two rude rocks. The three visionary girls are likewise there. In the deepening twilight, while the surf is dashing near their hearth, the ruddy gleam of the fire throws a strange air of comfort over the wild cove, bestrewn as it is with pebbles and sea-weed, and exposed to the "melancholy main." Moreover, as the smoke climbs up the precipice, it brings with it a savory smell from a pan of fried fish, and a black kettle of chowder, and reminds me that my dinner was nothing but bread and water, and a tuft of samphire, and an apple. Methinks the party might find room for another guest, at that flat rock which serves them for a table; and if spoons be scarce, I could pick up a clamshell on the beach. They see me now; and—the blessing of a hungry man upon him!—one of them sends up a hospitable shout—halloo, Sir Solitary! come down and sup with us! The ladies wave their handkerchiefs. Can I decline? No; and be it owned, after all my solitary joys, that this is the sweetest moment of a Day by the Sea-Shore.

Richard Long
A FOUR DAY WALK

A LINE OF GROUND 94 MILES LONG

ROAD   STONY TRACK ROAD GRASS FIELD
ROAD   BARE ROCK LANE ROAD STONY PATH
HEATHER BURNT MOOR STONY PATH ROAD
ROUGH GRASSLAND RIVERBED SHEEPTRACKS EARTH WALL
ROUGH GRASSLAND GRASS FIELDS BRAMBLES GRASS FIELD
ROAD WOODLAND PATH ROAD DUSTY LANE
ROAD GRASS FIELDS EARTH PATH ROAD
SAND BEACH CLIFF PATH ROAD ROCKS
CLIFF PATH SAND DUNES SAND PATH EARTH PATH
ROAD OLD RAILWAY TRACK MUD FLATS SEA WALL
MUD FLATS ROAD RIVERBANK ROAD

Max Beerbohm
GOING OUT FOR A WALK

It is a fact that not once in all my life have I gone out for walk. I have been taken out for walks; but that is another matter. Even while I trotted prattling by my nurse's side I regretted the good old days when I had, and wasn't, a perambulator. When I grew up it seemed to me that the one advantage of living in London was that nobody ever wanted me to come out for a walk. London's very drawbacks—its endless noise and bustle, its smoky air, the squalor ambushed everywhere in it—assured this one immunity. Whenever I was with friends in the country, I knew that at any moment, unless rain were actually falling, some man might suddenly say "Come out for a walk!" in that sharp imperative tone which he would not dream of using in any other connexion. People seem to think there is something inherently noble and virtuous in the desire to go for a walk. Any one thus desirous feels that he has a right to impose his will on whomever he sees comfortably settled in an arm-chair, reading. It is easy to say simply "No" to an old friend. In the case of a mere acquaintance one wants some excuse. "I wish I could, but"—nothing ever occurs to me except "I have some letters to write." This formula is unsatisfactory in three ways. (1) It isn't believed. (2) It compels you to rise from your chair, go to the writing-table, and sit improvising a letter to somebody until the walkmonger (just not daring to call you liar and hypocrite) shall have lumbered out of the room. (3) It won't operate on Sunday mornings. "There's no post out till this evening" clinches the matter; and you may as well go quietly.

Walking for walking's sake may be as highly laudable and exemplary a thing as it is held to be by those who practise it. My objection to it is that it stops the brain. Many a man has professed to me that his brain never works so well as when he is swinging along the high road or over hill and dale. This boast is not confirmed by my memory of anybody who on a Sunday morning has forced me to partake of his adventure. Experience teaches me that whatever a fellow-guest may have of power to instruct or to amuse when he is sitting on a chair, or standing on a hearth-rug, quickly leaves him when he takes one out for a walk. The ideas that came so thick and fast to him in any room, where are they now? where that encyclopaedic knowledge which he bore so lightly? where the kindling fancy that played like summer lightning over *any* topic that was started? The man's face that was so mobile is set now; gone is the light from his fine eyes. He says that A. (our host) is a thoroughly good fellow. Fifty yards further on, he adds that A. is one of the best fellows he has ever met. We tramp another furlong or so, and he says that Mrs. A. is a charming woman. Presently he adds that she is one of the most charming women he has ever known. We pass an inn. He reads vapidly aloud to me: "The Kings Arms. Licensed to sell Ales and Spirits." I foresee that during the rest of the walk he will read aloud any inscription that occurs. We pass a milestone. He points at it with his stick, and says "Uxminster. 11 miles." We turn a sharp corner at the foot of a hill. He points at the wall, and says "Drive Slowly." I see far ahead, on the other side of the hedge bordering the high road, a small notice-board. He sees it too. He keeps his eye on it. And in due course "Trespassers," he says, "Will Be Prosecuted." Poor man!—mentally a wreck.

Luncheon at the A.s, however, salves him and floats him in full sail. Behold him once more the life and soul of the party. Surely he will never, after the bitter lesson of this morning, go out for another walk. An hour later, I see him striding forth, with a new companion. I watch him out of sight. I know what he is saying. He is saying that I am rather a dull man to go a walk with. He will presently add that I am one of the dullest men he ever went a walk with. Then he will devote himself to reading out the inscriptions.

How comes it, this immediate deterioration in those who go walking for walking's sake? Just what happens? I take it that not by his reasoning faculties is a man urged to this enterprise. He is urged, evidently, by something in him that transcends reason; by his soul, I presume. Yes, it must be the soul that raps out the "Quick march!" to the body.—"Halt! Stand at ease!" interposes the brain, and "To what destination," it suavely asks the soul, "and on what errand, are you sending the body?" —"On no errand whatsoever," the soul makes answer, "and to no destination at all. It is just like you to be always on the look-out for some subtle ulterior motive. The body is going out because the mere fact of its doing so is a sure indication of nobility, probity, and rugged grandeur of character."—"Very well, Vagula, have your own wayula! But I," says the brain, "flatly refuse to be mixed up in this tomfoolery. I shall go to sleep till it is over." The brain then wraps itself up in its own convolutions, and falls into a dreamless slumber from which nothing can rouse it till the body has been safely deposited indoors again.

Even if you go to some definite place, for some definite purpose, the brain would rather you took a vehicle; but it does not make a point of this; it will serve you well enough unless you are going *out for a walk*. It won't, while your legs are vying with each other, do any deep thinking for you, nor even any close thinking; but it will do any number of small odd jobs for you willingly— provided that your legs, also, are making themselves useful, not merely bandying you about to gratify the pride of the soul. Such as it is, this essay was composed in the course of a walk, this morning. I am not one of those extremists who must have a vehicle to every destination. I never go out of my way, as it were, to avoid exercise. I take it as it comes, and take it in good part. That valetudinarians are always chattering about it, and indulging in it to excess, is no reason for despising it. I am inclined to think that in moderation it is rather good for one, physically. But, pending a time when no people wish me to go and see them, and I have no wish to go and see any one, and there is nothing whatever for me to do off my own premises, I never will go out for a walk.

Dorothy Wordsworth
FROM THE GRASMERE JOURNALS

April 15th, Thursday.—It was a threatening, misty morning, but mild. We set off after dinner from Eusemere. Mrs. Clarkson went a short way with us, but turned back. The wind was furious, and we thought we must have returned. We first rested in the large boathouse, then under a furze bush opposite Mr. Clarkson's. Saw the plough going in the field. The wind seized our breath. The lake was rough. There was a boat by itself floating in the middle of the bay below Water Millock. We rested again in the Water Millock Lane. The hawthorns are black and green, the birches here and there greenish, but there is yet more of purple to be seen on the twigs. We got over into a field to avoid some cows—people working. A few primroses by the roadside—woodsorrel flower, the anemone, scentless violets, strawberries, and that starry, yellow flower which Mrs. C. calls pile wort. When we were in the woods beyond Gowbarrow Park we saw a few daffodils close to the water-side. We fancied that the sea had floated the seeds ashore, and that the little colony had so sprung up. But as we went along there were more and yet more; and at last, under the boughs of the trees, we saw that there was a long belt of them along the shore, about the breadth of a country turnpike road. I never saw daffodils so beautiful. They grew among the mossy stones about and above them; some rested their heads on these stones, as on a pillow, for weariness; and the rest tossed and reeled and danced, and seemed as if they verily laughed with the wind, that blew upon them over the lake; they looked so gay, ever glancing, ever changing. This wind blew directly over the lake to them. There was here and there a little knot, and a few stragglers higher up; but they were so few as not to disturb the simplicity, unity, and life of that one busy highway. We rested again and again. The bays were stormy, and we heard the waves at different distances, and in the middle of the water, like the sea.

Walter Benjamin
HASHISH IN MARSEILLES

Preliminary remark: One of the first signs that hashish is beginning to take effect "is a dull feeling of foreboding; something strange, ineluctable is approaching . . . images and chains of images, long-submerged memories appear, whole scenes and situations are experienced; at first they arouse interest, now and then enjoyment, and finally, when there is no turning away from them, weariness and torment. By everything that happens, and by what he says and does, the subject is surprised and overwhelmed. His laughter, all his utterances happen to him like outward events. He also attains experiences that approach inspiration, illumination. . . . Space can expand, the ground tilt steeply, atmospheric sensations occur: vapor, an opaque heaviness of the air; colors grow brighter, more luminous; objects more beautiful, or else lumpy and threatening. . . . All this does not occur in a continuous development; rather, it is typified by a continual alternation of dreaming and waking states, a constant and finally exhausting oscillation between totally different worlds of consciousness; in the middle of a sentence these transitions can take place. . . . All this the subject reports in a form that usually diverges very widely from the norm. Connections become difficult to perceive, owing to the frequently sudden rupture of all memory of past events, thought is not formed into words, the situation can become so compulsively hilarious that the hashish eater for minutes on end is capable of nothing except laughing. . . . The memory of the intoxication is surprisingly clear." "It is curious that hashish poisoning has not yet been experimentally studied. The most admirable description of the hashish trance is by Baudelaire (*Les Paradis artificiels*)." From Joël and Fränkel, "Der Haschisch-Rausch," *Klinische Wochenschrift,* 1926, vol. 5, p. 37.

Marseilles, July 29. At seven o'clock in the evening, after long hesitation, I took hashish. During the day I had been in Aix. With the absolute certainty, in this city of hundreds of thousands where no one knows me, of not being disturbed, I lie on the bed. And yet I am disturbed, by a little child crying. I think three-quarters of an hour have already passed. But it is only twenty minutes. . . . So I lie on the bed, reading and smoking. Opposite me always this view of the belly of Marseilles. The street I have so often seen is like a knife cut.

At last I left the hotel, the effects seeming nonexistent or so weak that the precaution of staying at home was unnecessary. My first port of call was the café on the corner of Cannebière and Cours Belsunce. Seen from the harbor, the one on the right, therefore not my usual café. What now? Only a certain benevolence, the expectation of being received kindly by people. The feeling of loneliness is very quickly lost. My walking stick begins to give me a special pleasure. One becomes so tender, fears that a shadow falling on the paper might hurt it. The nausea disappears. One reads the notices on the urinals. It would not surprise me if this or that person came up to me. But when no one does I am not disappointed, either. However, it is too noisy for me here.

Now the hashish eater's demands on time and space come into force. As is known, these are absolutely regal. Versailles, for one who has taken hashish, is not too large, or eternity too long. Against the background of these immense dimensions of inner experience, of absolute duration and immeasurable space, a wonderful, beatific humor dwells all the more fondly on the contingencies of the world of space and time. I feel this humor infinitely when I am told at the Restaurant Basso that the hot kitchen has just been closed, while I have just sat down to feast into eternity. Afterward, despite this, the feeling that all this is indeed bright, frequented, animated, and will remain so. I must note how I found my seat. What mattered to me was the view of the old port that one got from the upper floors. Walking past below, I had spied an empty table on the balcony of the second story. Yet in the end I only reached the first. Most of the window tables were occupied, so I went up to a very large one that had just been vacated. As I was sitting down, however, the disproportion of seating myself at so large a table caused me such shame that I walked across the entire floor to the opposite end to sit at a smaller table that became visible to me only as I reached it.

But the meal came later. First, the little bar on the harbor. I was again just on the point of retreating in confusion, for a concert, indeed a brass band, seemed to be playing there. I only just managed to explain to myself that it was nothing more than the blaring of car horns. On the way to the Vieux Port I already had this wonderful lightness and sureness of step that transformed the stony, unarticulated earth of the great square that I was crossing into the surface of a country road along which I strode at night like an energetic hiker. For at this time I was still avoiding the Cannebière, not yet quite sure of my regulatory functions. In that little harbor bar the hashish then began to exert its canonical magic with a primitive sharpness that I had scarcely felt until then. For it made me into a physiognomist, or at least a contemplator of physiognomies, and I underwent something unique in my experience: I positively fixed my gaze on the faces that I had around me, which were, in part, of remarkable coarseness or ugliness. Faces that I would normally have avoided for a twofold reason: I should neither have wished to attract their gaze nor endured their brutality. It was a very advanced post, this harbor tavern. (I believe it was the farthest accessible to me without danger, a circumstance I had gauged, in the trance, with the same accuracy with which, when utterly weary, one is able to fill a glass exactly to the brim without spilling a drop, as one can never do with sharp senses.) It was still sufficiently far from rue Bouterie, yet no bourgeois sat there; at the most, besides the true port proletariat, a few petit-bourgeois families from the neighborhood. I now suddenly understood how, to a painter—had it not happened to Rembrandt and many others?—ugliness could appear as the true reservoir of beauty, better than any treasure cask, a jagged mountain with all the inner gold of beauty gleaming from the wrinkles, glances, features. I especially remember a boundlessly animal and vulgar male face in which the "line of renunciation" struck me with sudden violence. It was above all men's faces that had begun to interest me. Now began the game, to be long maintained, of recognizing someone I knew in every face; often I knew the name, often not; the deception vanished as deceptions vanish in dreams: not in shame and compromised, but peacefully and amiably, like a being who has performed his service. Under these circumstances there was no question of loneliness. Was I my own company? Surely not so undisguisedly. I doubt whether that would have made me so happy. More likely this: I became my own most skillful, fond, shameless procurer, gratifying myself with the ambiguous assurance of one who knows from profound study the wishes of his employer. Then it began to take half an eternity until the waiter reappeared. Or, rather, I could not wait for him to appear. I went into the barroom and paid at the counter. Whether tips are usual in such taverns I do not know. But under other circumstances I should have given something in any case. Under hashish yesterday, however, I was on the stingy side; for fear of attracting attention by extravagance, I succeeded in making myself really conspicuous.

Similarly at Basso's. First I ordered a dozen oysters. The man wanted me to order the next course at the same time. I named some local dish. He came back with the news that none was left. I then pointed to a place in the menu in the vicinity of this dish, and was on the point of ordering each item, one after another, but then the name of the one above it caught my attention, and so on, until I finally reached the top of the list. This was not just from greed, however, but from an extreme politeness toward the dishes that I did not wish to offend by a refusal. In short, I came to a stop at a *pâté de Lyon*. Lion paste, I thought with a witty smile, when it lay clean on a plate before me, and then, contemptuously: This tender rabbit or chicken meat—whatever it may be. To my lionish hunger it would not have seemed inappropriate to satisfy itself on a lion. Moreover, I had tacitly decided that as soon as I had finished at Basso's (it was about half past ten) I should go elsewhere and dine a second time.

But first, back to the walk to Basso's. I strolled along the quay and read one after another the names of the boats tied up there. As I did so an incomprehensible gaiety came over me, and I smiled in turn at all the Christian names of France. The love promised to these boats by their names seemed wonderfully beautiful and touching to me. Only one of them, Aero II, which reminded me of aerial warfare, I passed by without cordiality, exactly as, in the bar that I had just left, my gaze had been obliged to pass over certain excessively deformed countenances.

Upstairs at Basso's, when I looked down, the old games began again. The square in front of the harbor was my palette, on which imagination mixed the qualities of the place, trying them out now this way, now that, without concern for the result, like a painter daydreaming on his palette. I hesitated before taking wine. It was a half bottle of Cassis. A piece of ice was floating in the glass. Yet it went excellently with my drug. I had chosen my seat on account of the open window, through which I could look down on the dark square. And as I did so from time to time, I noticed that it had a tendency to change with everyone who stepped onto it, as if it formed a figure about him that, clearly, had nothing to do with the square as he saw it but, rather, with the view that the great portrait painters of the seventeenth century, in accordance with the character of the dignitary whom they placed before a colonnade or a window, threw into a relief by this colonnade, this window. Later I noted as I looked down, "From century to century things grow more estranged."

Here I must observe in general: the solitude of such trances has its dark side. To speak only of the physical aspect, there was a moment in the harbor tavern when a violent pressure in the diaphragm sought relief through humming. And there is no doubt that truly beautiful, illuminating visions were not awakened. On the other hand, solitude works in these states as a filter. What one writes down the following day is more than an enumeration of impressions; in the night the trance cuts itself off from everyday reality with fine, prismatic edges; it forms a kind of figure and is more easily memorable. I should like to say: it shrinks and takes on the form of a flower.

To begin to solve the riddle of the ecstasy of trance, one ought to meditate on Ariadne's thread. What joy in the mere act of unrolling a ball of thread. And this joy is very deeply related to the joy of trance, as to that of creation. We go forward; but in so doing we not only discover the twists and turns of the cave, but also enjoy this pleasure of discovery against the background of the other, rhythmical bliss of unwinding the thread. The certainty of unrolling an artfully wound skein—is that not the joy of all productivity, at least in prose? And under hashish we are enraptured prose-beings in the highest power.

A deeply submerged feeling of happiness that came over me afterward, on a square off the Cannebière where rue Paradis opens onto a park, is more difficult to recall than everything that went before. Fortunately I find on my newspaper the sentence "One should scoop sameness from reality with a spoon." Several weeks earlier I had noted another, by Johannes V. Jensen, which appeared to say something similar: "Richard was a young man with understanding for everything in the world that was of the same kind." This sentence had pleased me very much. It enabled me now to confront the political, rational sense it had had for me earlier with the individual, magical meaning of my experience the day before. Whereas Jensen's sentence amounted, as I had understood it, to saying that things are as we know them to be, thoroughly mechanized and rationalized, the particular being confined today solely to nuances, my new insight was entirely different. For I saw only nuances, yet these were the same. I immersed myself in contemplation of the sidewalk before me, which, through a kind of unguent with which I covered it, could have been, precisely as these very stones, also the sidewalk of Paris. One often speaks of stones instead of bread. These stones were the bread of my imagination, which was suddenly seized by a ravenous hunger to taste what is the same in all places and countries. And yet I thought with immense pride of sitting here in Marseilles in a hashish trance; of who else might be sharing my intoxication this evening, how few. Of how I was incapable of fearing future misfortune, future solitude, for hashish would always remain. The music from a nearby nightclub that I had been following played a part in this stage. G. rode past me in a cab. It happened suddenly, exactly as, earlier, from the shadows of the boat, U. had suddenly detached himself in the form of a harbor loafer and pimp. But there were not only known faces. Here, while I was in the state of deepest trance, two figures—citizens, vagrants, what do I know?—passed me as "Dante and Petrarch." "All men are brothers." So began a train of thought that I am no longer able to pursue. But its last link was certainly much less banal than its first and led on perhaps to images of animals.

"Barnabe," read the sign on a streetcar that stopped briefly at the square where I was sitting. And the sad confused story of Barnabas seemed to me no bad destination for a streetcar going into the outskirts of Marseilles. Something very beautiful was going on around the door of the dance hall. Now and then a Chinese in blue silk trousers and a glowing pink silk jacket stepped outside. He was the doorman. Girls displayed themselves in the doorway. My mood was free of all desire. It was amusing to see a young man with a girl in a white dress coming toward me and to be immediately obliged to think: "She got away from him in there in her shift, and now he is fetching her back. Well, well." I felt flattered by the thought of sitting here in a center of dissipation, and by "here" I did not mean the town but the little, not-very-eventful spot where I found myself. But events took place in such a way that the appearance of things touched me with a magic wand, and I sank into a dream of them. People and things behave at such hours like those little stage sets and people made of elder pith in the glazed tin-foil box, which, when the glass is rubbed, are electrified and fall at every movement into the most unusual relationships.

The music that meanwhile kept rising and falling, I called the rush switches of jazz. I have forgotten on what grounds I permitted myself to mark the beat with my foot. This is against my education, and it did not happen without inner disputation. There were times when the intensity of acoustic impressions blotted out all others. In the little bar, above all, everything was suddenly submerged in the noise of voices, not of streets. What was most peculiar about this din of voices was that it sounded entirely like dialect. The people of Marseilles suddenly did not speak good enough French for me. They were stuck at the level of dialect. The phenomenon of alienation that may be involved in this, which Kraus has formulated in the fine dictum "The more closely you look at a word the more distantly it looks back," appears to extend to the optical. At any rate I find among my notes the surprised comment "How things withstand the gaze."

The trance abated when I crossed the Cannebière and at last turned the corner to have a final ice cream at the little Café des Cours Belsunce. It was not far from the first café of the evening, in which, suddenly, the amorous joy dispensed by the contemplation of some fringes blown by the wind had convinced me that the hashish had begun its work. And when I recall this state I should like to believe that hashish persuades nature to permit us—for less egoistic purposes—that squandering of our own existence that we know in love. For if, when we love, our existence runs through nature's fingers like golden coins that she cannot hold and lets fall to purchase new birth thereby, she now throws us, without hoping or expecting anything, in ample handfuls to existence.

Christina Rossetti
THE HILLS ARE TIPPED WITH SUNSHINE, WHILE I WALK

The hills are tipped with sunshine, while I walk
   In shadows dim and cold:
The unawakened rose sleeps on her stalk
   In a bud's fold,
     Until the sun flood all the world with gold.

The hills are crowned with glory, and the glow
   Flows widening down apace:
Unto the sunny hilltops I, set low,
   Lift a tired face—
     Ah, happy rose, content to wait for grace!

How tired a face, how tired a brain, how tired
   A heart I lift, who long
For something never felt but still desired;
   Sunshine and song,
Song where the choirs of sunny heaven stand choired.

Gerard Manley Hopkins
HURRAHING IN HARVEST

Summer ends now; now, barbarous in beauty, the stooks arise
  Around; up above, what wind-walks! what lovely behaviour
  Of silk-sack clouds! has wilder, wilful-wavier
Meal-drift moulded ever and melted across skies?

I walk, I lift up, I lift up heart, eyes,
  Down all that glory in the heavens to glean our Saviour;
  And, éyes, heárt, what looks, what lips yet gave you a
Rapturous love's greeting of realer, of rounder replies?

And the azurous hung hills are his world-wielding shoulder
  Majestic—as a stallion stalwart, very-violet-sweet!—
These things, these things were here and but the beholder
  Wanting; which two when they once meet,
The heart réars wíngs bold and bolder
  And hurls for him, O half hurls earth for him off under his feet.

Emily Dickinson
I STEPPED FROM PLANK TO PLANK

I stepped from Plank to Plank
A slow and cautious way
The Stars about my Head I felt
About my Feet the Sea.

I knew not but the next
Would be my final inch—
This gave me that precarious Gait
Some call Experience.

Henry Vaughan
I WALK'D THE OTHER DAY

I walk'd the other day, to spend my hour,
   Into a field,
Where I sometimes had seen the soil to yield
   A gallant flow'r;
But winter now had ruffled all the bow'r
   And curious store
   I knew there heretofore.

Yet I, whose search lov'd not to peep and peer
   I' th' face of things,
Thought with my self, there might be other springs
   Besides this here,
Which, like cold friends, sees us but once a year;
   And so the flow'r
   Might have some other bow'r.

Then taking up what I could nearest spy,
   I digg'd about
That place where I had seen him to grow out;
   And by and by
I saw the warm recluse alone to lie,
   Where fresh and green
   He liv'd of us unseen.

Many a question intricate and rare
   Did I there strow;
But all I could extort was, that he now
   Did there repair

Such losses as befell him in this air,
  And would ere long
  Come forth most fair and young.

This past, I threw the clothes quite o'er his head;
  And stung with fear
Of my own frailty dropp'd down many a tear
  Upon his bed;
Then sighing whisper'd, "happy are the dead!
  What peace doth now
  Rock him asleep below!"

And yet, how few believe such doctrine springs
  From a poor root,
Which all the winter sleeps here under foot,
  And hath no wings
To raise it to the truth and light of things;
  But is still trod
  By ev'ry wand'ring clod.

O Thou! whose spirit did at first inflame
  And warm the dead,
And by a sacred incubation fed
  With life this frame,
Which once had neither being, form, nor name;
  Grant I may so
  Thy steps track here below,

That in these masques and shadows I may see
  Thy sacred way;
And by those hid ascents climb to that day,
  Which breaks from Thee,
Who art in all things, though invisibly!
  Shew me thy peace,
  Thy mercy, love, and ease,

And from this care, where dreams and sorrows reign,
   Lead me above,
Where light, joy, leisure, and true comforts move
   Without all pain;
There, hid in thee, shew me his life again,
   At whose dumb urn
   Thus all the year I mourn.

William Wordsworth
I WANDERED LONELY AS A CLOUD

I wandered lonely as a cloud
That floats on high o'er vales and hills,
When all at once I saw a crowd,
A host, of golden daffodils;
Beside the lake, beneath the trees,
Fluttering and dancing in the breeze.

Continuous as the stars that shine
And twinkle on the milky way,
They stretched in never-ending line
Along the margin of a bay:
Ten thousand saw I at a glance,
Tossing their heads in sprightly dance.

The waves beside them danced; but they
Out-did the sparkling waves in glee:
A poet could not but be gay,
In such a jocund company:
I gazed—and gazed—but little thought
What wealth the show to me had brought:

For oft, when on my couch I lie
In vacant or in pensive mood,
They flash upon that inward eye
Which is the bliss of solitude;
And then my heart with pleasure fills,
And dances with the daffodils.

Ralph Waldo Emerson
FROM JOURNALS

July 1828

It is a peculiarity (I find by observation upon others) of humour in me, my strong propensity for strolling. I deliberately shut up my books in a cloudy July noon, put on my old clothes & old hat & slink away to the whortleberry bushes & slip with the greatest satisfaction into a little cowpath where I am sure I can defy observation. This point gained, I solace myself for hours with picking blueberries & other trash of the woods far from fame behind the birch trees. I seldom enjoy hours as I do these. I remember them in winter; I expect them in spring. I do not know a creature that I think has the same humour or would think it respectable. . . .

April 11, 1834

Went yesterday to Cambridge and spent most of the day at Mount Auburn; got my luncheon at Fresh Pond, and went back again to the woods. After much wandering and seeing many things, four snakes gliding up and down a hollow for no purpose that I could see—not to eat, not for love, but only gliding; then a whole bed of *Hepatica triloba,* cousins of the Anemone, all blue and beautiful, but constrained by niggard nature to wear their last year's faded jacket of leaves; then a black-capped titmouse, who came upon a tree, and when I would know his name, sang *chick-a-dee-dee;* then a far-off tree full of clamorous birds, I know not what, but you might hear them half a mile; I forsook the tombs, and found a sunny hollow where the east wind would not blow, and lay down against the side of a tree to most happy beholdings. At last I opened my eyes and let what would pass through them into the soul. I saw no more my relation, how near and petty, to Cambridge or Boston; I heeded no more what minute or hour our Massachusetts clocks might indicate—I saw only the noble earth on which I was born, with the great Star which warms and enlightens it. I saw the clouds that hang their significant drapery over us. It was Day—that was all Heaven said. The pines glittered with their innumerable green needles in the light, and seemed to challenge me to read their riddle. The drab oak-leaves of the last year turned their little somersets and lay still again. And the wind bustled high overhead in the forest top. This gay and grand architecture, from the vault to the moss and lichen on which I lay,—who shall explain to me the laws of its proportions and adornments?

May 11, 1838

Last night the moon rose behind four distinct pine-tree tops in the distant woods and the night at ten was so bright that I walked abroad. But the sublime light of night is unsatisfying, provoking; it astonishes but explains not. Its charm floats, dances, disappears, comes and goes, but palls in five minutes after you have left the house. Come out of your warm, angular house, resounding with few voices, into the chill, grand, instantaneous night, with such a Presence as a full moon in the clouds, and you are struck with poetic wonder. In the instant you leave far behind all human relations, wife, mother and child, and live only with the savages—water, air, light, carbon, lime, and granite. I think of Kuhleborn. I become a moist, cold element. 'Nature grows over me.' Frogs pipe; waters far off tinkle; dry leaves hiss; grass bends and rustles, and I have died out of the human world and come to feel a strange, cold, aqueous, terraqueous, aerial, ethereal sympathy and existence. I sow the sun and moon for seeds.

June 28, 1838

The moon and Jupiter side by side last night stemmed the sea of clouds and plied their voyage in convoy through the sublime Deep as I walked the old and dusty road. The snow and the enchantment of the moonlight make all landscapes alike, and the road that is so tedious and homely that I never take it by day, —by night is Italy or Palmyra. In these divine pleasures permitted to me of walks in the June night under moon and stars, I can put my life as a fact before me and stand aloof from its honor and shame.

John Clare
JOURNEY OUT OF ESSEX

July 18—1841—Sunday—Felt very melancholly—went a walk on the forest
in the afternoon—fell in with some gipseys one of whom offered to assist in
my escape from the mad house by hideing me in his camp to which I almost
agreed but told him I had no money to start with but if he would do so I
would promise him fifty pounds and he agreed to do so before saturday   on
friday I went again but he did not seem so willing so I said little about it—On
sunday I went and they were all gone—an old wide awake hat and an old
straw bonnet of the plumb pudding sort was left behind—and I put the hat in
my pocket thinking it might be usefull for another oppertunity—as good luck
would have it, it turned out to be so

July 19—Monday—Did nothing

July 20—Reconnitered the rout the Gipsey pointed out and found it a legi-
ble one to make a movement and having only honest courage and myself in
my army I Led the way and my troops soon followed but being careless in
mapping down the rout as the Gipsey told me I missed the lane to Enfield
town and was going down Enfield highway till I passed 'The Labour in vain'
Public house where A person I knew comeing out of the door told me the way
   I walked down the lane gently and was soon in Enfield Town and bye and
bye on the great York Road where it was all plain sailing and steering ahead
meeting no enemy and fearing none I reached Stevenage where being Night I
got over a gate crossed over the corner of a green paddock where seeing a pond
or hollow in the corner I forced to stay off a respectable distance to keep from
falling into it for my legs were nearly knocked up and began to stagger   I
scaled some old rotten paleings into the yard and then had higher pailings to
clamber over to get into the shed or hovel which I did with difficulty being
rather weak and to my good luck I found some trusses of clover piled up about

6 or more feet square which I gladly mounted and slept on   there was some trays in the hovel on which I could have reposed had I not found a better bed

I slept soundly but had a very uneasy dream I thought my first wife lay on my left arm and somebody took her away from my side which made me wake up rather unhappy I thought as I awoke somebody said 'Mary' but nobody was near—I lay down with my head towards the north to show myself the steering point in the morning

July 21—[when I awoke] Daylight was looking in on every side and fearing my garrison might be taken by storm and myself be made prisoner I left my lodging by the way I got in and thanked God for his kindness in procureing it (for any thing in a famine is better then nothing and any place that giveth the weary rest is a blessing)   I gained the north road again and steered due north—on the left hand side the road under the bank like a cave I saw a Man and boy coiled up asleep which I hailed and they woke up to tell me the name of the next village

Some where on the London side the 'Plough' Public house a Man passed me on horseback in a Slop frock and said 'here's another of the broken down haymakers' and threw me a penny to get a half pint of beer which I picked up and thanked him for and when I got to the plough I called for a half pint and drank it and got a rest and escaped a very heavy shower in the bargain by having a shelter till it was over—afterwards I would have begged a penny of two drovers who were very saucey so I begged no more of any body meet who I would

—I passed 3 or 4 good built houses on a hill and a public house on the road side in the hollow below them   I seemed to pass the Milestones very quick in the morning but towards night they seemed to be stretched further asunder I got to a village further on and forgot the name   the road on the left hand was quite over shaded by some trees and quite dry so I sat down half an hour and made a good many wishes for breakfast but wishes was no hearty meal so I got up as hungry as I sat down—I forget here the names of the villages I passed through but reccolect at late evening going through Potton in Bedfordshire where I called in a house to light my pipe in which was a civil old woman and a young country wench makeing lace on a cushion as round as a globe and a young fellow all civil people—I asked them a few questions as to the way and where the clergyman and overseer lived but they scarcely heard me or gave me no answer

I then went through Potton and happened with a kind talking country man who told me the Parson lived a good way from where I was or overseer I do'n't know which so I went on hopping with a crippled foot for the gravel had got into my old shoes one of which I had now nearly lost the sole   Had I found the overseers house at hand or the Parsons I should have gave my name and begged for a shilling to carry me home but I was forced to brush on pennyless and be thankfull I had a leg to move on—I then asked him wether he could tell me of a farm yard any where on the road where I could find a shed and some dry straw and he said yes and if you will go with me I will show you the place—its a public house on the left hand side the road at the sign of the 'Ram' but seeing a stone or flint heap I longed to rest as one of my feet was very painfull so I thanked him for his kindness and bid him go on—but the good natured fellow lingered awhile as if wishing to conduct me and then suddenly reccolecting that he had a hamper on his shoulder and a lock up bag in his hand cram full to meet the coach which he feared missing—he started hastily and was soon out of sight—I followed looking in vain for the country mans straw bed—and not being able to meet it I lay down by a shed side under some Elm trees between the wall and the trees being a thick row planted some 5 or 6 feet from the buildings   I lay there and tried to sleep but the wind came in between them so cold that I lay till I quaked like the ague and quitted the lodging for a better at the Ram which I could hardly hope to find—It now began to grow dark apace and the odd houses on the road began to light up and show the inside tennants lots very comfortable and my outside lot very uncomfortable and wretched—still I hobbled forward as well as I could and at last came to the Ram   the shutters were not closed and the lighted window looked very cheering but I had no money and did not like to go in

there was a sort of shed or gighouse at the end but I did not like to lie there as the people were up—so I still travelled on   the road was very lonely and dark in places being overshaded with trees   at length I came to a place where the road branched off into two turnpikes one to the right about and the other straight forward and on going bye my eye glanced on a mile stone standing under the hedge so I heedlessly turned back to read it to see where the other road led too and on doing so I found it led to London   I then suddenly forgot which was North or South and though I narrowly examined both ways I could see no tree or bush or stone heap that I could reccolect I had passed so I went on mile after mile almost convinced I was going the same way I came and these thoug[h]ts were so strong upon me that doubt and hopelessness made me turn so feeble that I was scarcely able to walk yet I could not sit down or give up but shuffled along till I saw a lamp shining as bright as the moon which on nearing I found was suspended over a Tollgate   before I got through the man came out with a candle and eyed me narrowly but having no fear I stopt to ask him wether I was going northward and he said when you get through the gate you are; so I thanked him kindly and went through on the other side and gathered my old strength   as my doubts vanished I soon cheered up and hummed the air of highland Mary as I went on   I at length fell in with an odd house all alone near a wood but I could not see what the sign was though the sign seemed to stand oddly enough in a sort of trough or spout   there was a large porch over the door and being weary I crept in and glad enough I was to find I could lye with my legs straight   the inmates were all gone to roost for I could hear them turn over in bed as I lay at full length on the stones in the poach—I slept here till daylight and felt very much refreshed as I got up—I blest my two wives and both their familys when I lay down and when I got up and when I thought of some former difficultys on a like occasion I could not help blessing the Queen   Having passed a Lodge on the left hand within a mile and half or less of a town I think it might be St Ives but I forget the name I sat down to rest on a flint heap where I might rest half an hour or more and while sitting here I saw a tall Gipsey come out of the Lodge gate and make down the road towards where I was sitting   when she got up to me on seeing she was a young woman with an honest looking countenance rather handsome I spoke to her and asked her a few questions which she answered readily and with evident good humor so I got up and went on to the next town with her—she cautioned me on the way to put somthing in my hat to keep the crown up and said in a lower tone 'you'll be noticed' but not knowing what she hinted—I took no notice and made no reply   at length she pointed to a small tower church which she called Shefford Church and advised me to go on a footway which would take me direct to it and I should shorten my journey fifteen miles by doing so   I would gladly have taken the young womans advice feeling that it was honest and a nigh guess towards the truth but fearing I might loose my way and not be able to find the north road again I thanked her and told her I should keep to the road when she bade me 'good day' and went into a house or shop on the left hand side the road   I have but a slight reccolection of my journey between here and Stilton for I was knocked up and noticed little or nothing—one night I lay in a dyke bottom from the wind and went sleep half an hour when I suddenly awoke and found one side wet through from the sock in the dyke bottom so I got out and went on—I remember going down a very dark road hung over with trees on both sides very thick which seemed to extend a mile or two   I then entered a town and some of the chamber windows had candle lights shineing in them—I felt so weak here that I forced to sit down on the ground to rest myself and while I sat her a Coach that seemed to be heavy laden came rattling up and stopt in the hollow below me and I cannot reccolect its ever passing by me   I then got up and pushed onward seeing little to notice for the road very often looked as stupid as myself and I was very often half asleep as I went   on the third day I satisfied my hunger by eating the grass by the road side which seemed to taste something like bread   I was hungry and eat heartily till I was satisfied and in fact the meal seemed to do me good   the next and last day I reccollected that I had some tobacco and my box of lucifers being exausted I could not light my pipe so I took to chewing Tobacco all day and eat the quids when I had done and I was never hungry afterwards—I remember passing through Buckden and going a length of road afterwards but I dont reccolect the name of any place untill I came to stilton where I was compleatly foot foundered and bro-ken down   when I had got about half through the town a gravel causeway invited me to rest myself so I lay down and nearly went sleep   a young woman (so I guessed by the voice) came out of a house and said 'poor creature' and another more elderly said 'O he shams' but when I got up the latter said 'o no he don't' as I hobbled along very lame   I heard the voices but never looked back to see where they came from—when I got near the Inn at the end of the gravel walk I met two young women and I asked one of them wether the road branching to the right bye the end of the Inn did not lead to Peterborough and she said 'Yes' it did so as soon as ever I was on it I felt myself in homes way and went on rather more cheerfull though I forced to rest oftener then usual

before I got to Peterborough a man and woman passed me in a cart and on hailing me as they passed I found they were neighbours from Helpstone where I used to live—I told them I was knocked up which they could easily see and that I had neither eat or drank any thing since I left Essex   when I told my story they clubbed together and threw me fivepence out of the cart   I picked it up and called at a small public house near the bridge were I had two half pints of ale and twopenn'oth of bread and cheese   when I had done I started quite refreshed only my feet was more crippled then ever and I could scarcely make a walk of it over the stones and being half ashamed to sit down in the street I forced to keep on the move and got through Peterborough better then I expected   when I got on the high road I rested on the stone heaps as I passed till I was able to go on afresh and bye and bye I passed Walton and soon reached Werrington and was making for the Beehive as fast as I could when a cart met me with a man and woman and a boy in it when nearing me the woman jumped out and caught fast hold of my hands and wished me to get into the cart but I refused and thought her either drunk or mad but when I was told it was my second wife Patty I got in and was soon at Northborough

but Mary was not there neither could I get any information about her further then the old story of her being dead six years ago which might be taken from a bran new old Newspaper printed a dozen years ago but I took no notice of the blarney having seen her myself about a twelvemonth ago alive and well and as young as ever—so here I am homeless at home and half gratified to feet that I can be happy any where

'May none those marks of my sad fate efface
'For they appeal from tyranny to God'
        Byron

July 24th 1841 Returned home out of Essex and found no Mary—her and her family are as nothing to me now though she herself was once the dearest of all—and how can I forget

Hisieh Ling-Yun
JOURNEYING BY STREAM: FOLLOWING CHIN-CHU TORRENT I CROSS THE MOUNTAINS

Translated by Francis Westbrook

When the gibbons howl one is sure it's dawn,
Though in the valley gloom no light can be seen.
Beneath the cliffs clouds are just forming,
While on the flowers dewdrops still glisten.
Winding about through nook and crook,
I tortuously ascend to the notches and peaks.
Crossing streams I drench my clothes in the rapids,
Scaling cliff-ladders I traverse far spans.
The river's bank often doubles back;
I enjoy going with the meandering stream.
Duckweed floats on the murky depths,
Darnel and rushes cover the limpid shallows.

On tiptoe atop a stone I cup a waterfall,
And climbing a tree pull down leafy branches.
I fancy seeing someone in the mountain's fold:
The fig-leaf coat and rabbit-floss girdle are before my eyes.
Taking a handful of orchids, I try in vain to entwine them;
I break off hemp—to whom can I open my heart?
To my mind appreciation is beauty;
This thing is obscure—who can ever discern it?
Viewing this scenery I discard worldly cares;
Awakened once and for all, I'll gain total abandonment.

Simon Ortiz
LA JUNTA

La Junta:
        they let us
        be mad
in their town.

My partners, hollows
       and pockets,
are shadows
      of souls.
But souls nevertheless.

We park on a side street,
do not draw attention,
and wander away,
        shuffling.

I drift
   away
as shadow,

anonymous, not willing
to be mad.

     Nonetheless,
     nonetheless,
I am their partner. Them.

Thomas Hardy
THE LAST SIGNAL

(11 Oct. 1886)
A Memory of William Barnes

Silently I footed by an uphill road
That led from my abode to a spot yew-boughed;
Yellowly the sun sloped low down to westward,
          And dark was the east with cloud.

Then, amid the shadow of that livid sad east,
  Where the light was least, and a gate stood wide,
Something flashed the fire of the sun that was facing it,
          Like a brief blaze on that side.

Looking hard and harder I knew what it meant—
  The sudden shine sent from the livid east scene;
It meant the west mirrored by the coffin of my friend there,
          Turning to the road from his green,

To take his last journey forth—he who in his prime
  Trudged so many a time from that gate athwart the land!
Thus a farewell he signalled on his grave-way,
          As with a wave of his hand.

Winterborne-Came Path

John Keats

FROM LETTERS

To the George Keatses, 14 February–3 May 1819

. . . Last Sunday I took a Walk towards Highgate and in the lane that winds by the side of Lord Mansfield's park I met Mr Green our Demonstrator at Guy's in conversation with Coleridge—I joined them, after enquiring by a look whether it would be agreeable—I walked with him at his alderman-after-dinner pace for near two miles I suppose. In those two Miles he broached a thousand things—let me see if I can give you a list—Nightingales, Poetry—on Poetical sensation—Metaphysics—Different genera and species of Dreams —Nightmare—a dream accompanied by a sense of touch—single and double touch—A dream related—First and second consciousness—the difference explained between will and Volition—so many metaphysicians from a want of smoking the second consciousness—Monsters—the Kraken—Mermaids— Southey believes in them—Southey's belief too much diluted—A Ghost story—Good morning—I heard his voice as he came towards me—I heard it as he moved away—I had heard it all the interval—if it may be called so. He was civil enough to ask me to call on him at Highgate. Good night!

Robert Walser
A LITTLE RAMBLE

Translated by Tom Whalen

I walked through the mountains today. The weather was damp, and the entire region was gray. But the road was soft and in places very clean. At first I had my coat on; soon, however, I pulled it off, folded it together, and laid it upon my arm. The walk on the wonderful road gave me more and ever more pleasure; first it went up and then descended again. The mountains were huge, they seemed to go around. The whole mountainous world appeared to me like an enormous theater. The road snuggled up splendidly to the mountainsides. Then I came down into a deep ravine, a river roared at my feet, a train rushed past me with magnificent white smoke. The road went through the ravine like a smooth white stream, and as I walked on, to me it was as if the narrow valley were bending and winding around itself. Gray clouds lay on the mountains as though that were their resting place. I met a young traveler with a rucksack on his back, who asked if I had seen two other young fellows. No, I said. Had I come here from very far? Yes, I said, and went farther on my way. Not a long time, and I saw and heard the two young wanderers pass by with music. A village was especially beautiful with humble dwellings set thickly under the white cliffs. I encountered a few carts, otherwise nothing, and I had seen some children on the highway. We don't need to see anything out of the ordinary. We already see so much.

William Blake
LONDON

I wander thro' each charter'd street,
Near where the charter'd Thames does flow,
And mark in every face I meet
Marks of weakness, marks of woe.

In every cry of every Man,
In every Infant's cry of fear,
In every voice, in every ban,
The mind-forg'd manacles I hear.

How the Chimney-sweeper's cry
Every black'ning Church appalls;
And the hapless Soldier's sigh
Runs in blood down Palace walls.

But most thro' midnight streets I hear
How the youthful Harlot's curse
Blasts the new born Infant's tear,
And blights with plagues the Marriage hearse.

Robert Grenier
[A LONG WALK]

. . .

a long walk
a long
walk a long
walk a long
walk along

Ruth Stone
LOOKING FOR SIGNS

Charles and I turn right at the privet hedge.
We are six brisk feet stopping at random stations.
Alone on a porch, a baby behind bars
waves in a private language.
We have just moved in, 2nd floor, number 22.
We cross at the corner. No traffic except for birds.
This is an old established neighborhood.
Each lawn is mowed. Each driveway fresh asphalt.
It is Sunday; quiet as the color of washed blue.
Charles poops. We are embarrassed and walk on.

Street after street of silent well-kept houses,
embalmed with beds of marigolds, more explicit than words;
gratuitous designs of manicured slopes;
but, yes, a sweet disorderly fall of yellow leaves.
Thereupon, to the bells of nearby St. Blessed Ascension,
we pause at one aberrant yard with broken palings,
a house of uncurtained windows painted jonquil yellow,
to see from this angle the unlikely bodies
of three middle-aged cars jacked up on cement blocks
under the maples at the back,
where the uncut lawn is blessed with flowering weeds;
and although there is no one visible,
we are made strangely happy and walk on.

Henry David Thoreau
FROM THE MAINE WOODS

In the morning, after whetting our appetite on some raw pork, a wafer of hard bread, and a dipper of condensed cloud or water spout, we all together began to make our way up the falls, which I have described; this time choosing the right hand, or highest peak, which was not the one I had approached before. But soon my companions were lost to my sight behind the mountain ridge in my rear, which still seemed ever retreating before me, and I climbed alone over huge rocks, loosely poised, a mile or more, still edging toward the clouds—for though the day was clear elsewhere, the summit was concealed by mist. The mountain seemed a vast aggregation of loose rocks, as if sometime it had rained rocks, and they lay as they fell on the mountain sides, nowhere fairly at rest, but leaning on each other, all rocking-stones, with cavities between, but scarcely any soil or smoother shelf. They were the raw materials of a planet dropped from an unseen quarry, which the vast chemistry of nature would anon work up, or work down, into the smiling and verdant plains and valleys of earth. This was an undone extremity of the globe; as in lignite, we see coal in the process of formation.

At length I entered within the skirts of the cloud which seemed forever drifting over the summit, and yet would never be gone, but was generated out of that pure air as fast as it flowed away; and when, a quarter of a mile further, I reached the summit of the ridge, which those who have seen in clearer weather say is about five miles long, and contains a thousand acres of table-land, I was deep within the hostile ranks of clouds, and all objects were obscured by them. Now the wind would blow me out a yard of clear sunlight, wherein I stood; then a gray, dawning light was all it could accomplish, the cloud-line ever rising and falling with the wind's intensity. Sometimes it seemed as if the summit would be cleared in a few moments, and smile in sunshine: but what was gained on one side was lost on another. It was like sitting in a chimney and waiting for the smoke to blow away. It was, in fact, a cloud-factory,—these were the cloud-works, and the wind turned them off done from the cool, bare rocks. Occasionally, when the windy columns broke in to me, I caught sight of a dark, damp crag to the right or left; the mist driving ceaselessly between it and me. It reminded me of the creations of the old epic and dramatic poets, of Atlas, Vulcan, the Cyclops, and Prometheus. Such was Caucasus and the rock where Prometheus was bound. Æschylus had no doubt visited such scenery as this. It was vast, Titanic, and such as man never inhabits. Some part of the beholder, even some vital part, seems to escape through the loose grating of his ribs as he ascends. He is more lone than you can imagine. There is less of substantial thought and fair understanding in him, than in the plains where men inhabit. His reason is dispersed and shadowy, more thin and subtile, like the air. Vast, Titanic, inhuman Nature has got him at disadvantage, caught him alone, and pilfers him of some of his divine faculty. She does not smile on him as in the plains. She seems to say sternly, why came ye here before your time? This ground is not prepared for you. Is it not enough that I smile in the valleys? I have never made this soil for thy feet, this air for thy breathing, these rocks for thy neighbors. I cannot pity nor fondle thee here, but forever relentlessly drive thee hence to where I *am* kind. Why seek me where I have not called thee, and then complain because you find me but a stepmother? Shouldst thou freeze or starve, or shudder thy life away, here is no shrine, nor altar, nor any access to my ear.

> "Chaos and ancient Night, I come no spy
> With purpose to explore or to disturb
> The secrets of your realm, but . . .
> . . . . as my way
> Lies through your spacious empire up to light."

The tops of mountains are among the unfinished parts of the globe, whither it is a slight insult to the gods to climb and pry into their secrets, and try their effect on our humanity. Only daring and insolent men, perchance, go there. Simple races, as savages, do not climb mountains—their tops are sacred and mysterious tracts never visited by them. Pomola is always angry with those who climb to the summit of Ktaadn. . . .

Perhaps I most fully realized that this was primeval, untamed, and forever untameable *Nature,* or whatever else men call it, while coming down this part of the mountain. We were passing over "Burnt Lands," burnt by lightning, perchance, though they showed no recent marks of fire, hardly so much as a charred stump, but looked rather like a natural pasture for the moose and deer, exceedingly wild and desolate, with occasional strips of timber crossing them, and low poplars springing up, and patches of blueberries here and there. I found myself traversing them familiarly, like some pasture run to waste, or partially reclaimed by man; but when I reflected what man, what brother or sister or kinsman of our race made it and claimed it, I expected the proprietor to rise up and dispute my passage. It is difficult to conceive of a region uninhabited by man. We habitually presume his presence and influence everywhere. And yet we have not seen pure Nature, unless we have seen her thus vast, and drear, and inhuman, though in the midst of cities. Nature was here something savage and awful, though beautiful. I looked with awe at the ground I trod on, to see what the Powers had made there, the form and fashion and material of their work. This was that Earth of which we have heard, made out of Chaos and Old Night. Here was no man's garden, but the unhandselled globe. It was not lawn, nor pasture, nor mead, nor woodland, nor lea, nor arable, nor waste-land. It was the fresh and natural surface of the planet Earth, as it was made for ever and ever,—to be the dwelling of man, we say,—so Nature made it, and man may use it if he can. Man was not to be associated with it. It was Matter, vast, terrific,—not his Mother Earth that we have heard of, not for him to tread on, or be buried in,—no, it were being too familiar even to let his bones lie there,—the home this of Necessity and Fate. There was there felt the presence of a force not bound to be kind to man. It was a place for heathenism and superstitious rites,—to be inhabited by men nearer of kin to the rocks and to wild animals than we. We walked over it with a certain awe, stopping from time to time to pick the blueberries which grew there, and had a smart and spicy taste. Perchance where *our* wild pines stand, and leaves lie on their forest floor in Concord, there were once reapers, and husbandmen planted grain; but here not even the surface had been scarred by man, but it was a specimen of what God saw fit to make this world. What is it to be admitted to a museum, to see a myriad of particular things, compared with being shown some star's surface, some hard matter in its home! I stand in awe of my body, this matter to which I am bound has become so strange to me.

I fear not spirits, ghosts, of which I am one,—*that* my body might,—but I fear bodies, I tremble to meet them. What is this Titan that has possession of me? Talk of mysteries!—Think of our life in nature,—daily to be shown matter, to come in contact with it,—rocks, trees, wind on our cheeks! the *solid* earth! the actual world! the *common sense! Contact! Contact! Who* are we? *where* are we?

Edgar Allan Poe
THE MAN OF THE CROWD

Ce grand malheur, de ne pouvoir être seul.
—La Bruyère

It was well said of a certain German book that *"er lasst sich nicht lesen"*—it does not permit itself to be read. There are some secrets which do not permit themselves to be told. Men die nightly in their beds, wringing the hands of ghostly confessors, and looking them piteously in the eyes—die with despair of heart and convulsion of throat, on account of the hideousness of mysteries which will not *suffer themselves* to be revealed. Now and then, alas, the conscience of man takes up a burthen so heavy in horror that it can be thrown down only into the grave. And thus the essence of all crime is undivulged.

Not long ago, about the closing in of an evening in autumn, I sat at the large bow window of the D— Coffee-House in London. For some months I had been ill in health, but was now convalescent, and, with returning strength, found myself in one of those happy moods which are so precisely the converse of ennui—moods of the keenest appetency, when the film from the mental vision departs—the αχλυς ος πριν επηεν—and the intellect, electrified, surpasses as greatly its everyday condition, as does the vivid yet candid reason of Leibnitz, the mad and flimsy rhetoric of Gorgias. Merely to breathe was enjoyment; and I derived positive pleasure even from many of the legitimate sources of pain. I felt a calm but inquisitive interest in every thing. With a cigar in my mouth and a newspaper in my lap, I had been amusing myself for the greater part of the afternoon, now in poring over advertisements, now in observing the promiscuous company in the room, and now in peering through the smoky panes into the street.

This latter is one of the principal thoroughfares of the city, and had been very much crowded during the whole day. But, as the darkness came on, the throng momently increased; and, by the time the lamps were well lighted, two dense and continuous tides of population were rushing past the door. At this particular period of the evening I had never before been in a similar situation, and the tumultuous sea of human heads filled me, therefore, with a delicious novelty of emotion. I gave up, at length, all care of things within the hotel, and became absorbed in contemplation of the scene without.

At first my observations took an abstract and generalizing turn. I looked at the passengers in masses, and thought of them in their aggregate relations. Soon, however, I descended to details, and regarded with minute interest the innumerable varieties of figure, dress, air, gait, visage, and expression of countenance.

By far the greater number of those who went by had a satisfied, business-like demeanor, and seemed to be thinking only of making their way through the press. Their brows were knit, and their eyes rolled quickly; when pushed against by fellow-wayfarers they evinced no symptom of impatience, but adjusted their clothes and hurried on. Others, still a numerous class, were restless in their movements, had flushed faces, and talked and gesticulated to themselves, as if feeling in solitude on account of the very denseness of the company around. When impeded in their progress, these people suddenly ceased muttering, but redoubled their gesticulations, and awaited, with an absent and overdone smile upon the lips, the course of the persons impeding them. If jostled, they bowed profusely to the jostlers, and appeared overwhelmed with confusion. —There was nothing very distinctive about these two large classes beyond what I have noted. Their habiliments belonged to that order which is pointedly termed the decent. They were undoubtedly noblemen, merchants, attorneys, tradesmen, stock-jobbers—the Eupatrids and the common-places of society—men of leisure and men actively engaged in affairs of their own—conducting business upon their own responsibility. They did not greatly excite my attention.

The tribe of clerks was an obvious one and here I discerned two remarkable divisions. There were the junior clerks of flash houses—young gentlemen with tight coats, bright boots, well-oiled hair, and supercilious lips. Setting aside a certain dapperness of carriage, which may be termed *deskism* for want of a better word, the manner of these persons seemed to be an exact facsimile of what had been the perfection of *bon ton* about twelve or eighteen months before. They wore the cast-off graces of the gentry;—and this, I believe, involves the best definition of the class.

The division of the upper clerks of staunch firms, or of the "steady old fel-lows," it was not possible to mistake. These were known by their coats and pantaloons of black or brown, made to sit comfortably, with white cravats and waistcoats, broad solid-looking shoes, and thick hose or gaiters.—They had all slightly bald heads, from which the right ears, long used to penholding, had an odd habit of standing off on end. I observed that they always removed or set-tled their hats with both hands, and wore watches, with short gold chains of a substantial and ancient pattern. Theirs was the affectation of respectability;—if indeed there be an affectation so honorable.

There were many individuals of dashing appearance, whom I easily under-stood as belonging to the race of swell pick-pockets, with which all great cities are infested. I watched these gentry with much inquisitiveness, and found it difficult to imagine how they should ever be mistaken for gentlemen by gen-tlemen themselves. Their voluminousness of wristband, with an air of exces-sive frankness, should betray them at once.

The gamblers, of whom I descried not a few, were still more easily recog-nisable. They wore every variety of dress, from that of the desperate thimble-rig bully, with velvet waistcoat, fancy neckerchief, gilt chains, and filagreed buttons, to that of the scrupulously inornate clergyman, than which nothing could be less liable to suspicion. Still all were distinguished by a certain sodden swarthiness of complexion, a filmy dimness of eye, and pallor and compres-sion of lip. There were two other traits, moreover, by which I could always detect them;—a guarded lowness of tone in conversation, and a more than ordinary extension of the thumb in a direction at right angles with the fingers. Very often, in company with these sharpers, I observed an order of men some-what different in habits, but still birds of a kindred feather. They may be defined as the gentlemen who live by their wits. They seem to prey upon the public in two battalions—that of the dandies and that of the military men. Of the first grade the leading features are long locks and smiles; of the second frogged coats and frowns.

Descending in the scale of what is termed gentility, I found darker and deeper themes for speculation. I saw Jew pedlars, with hawk eyes flashing from countenances whose every other feature wore only an expression of abject humility; sturdy professional street beggars scowling upon mendicants of a better stamp, whom despair alone had driven forth into the night for charity; feeble and ghastly invalids, upon whom death had placed a sure hand, and who sidled and tottered through the mob, looking every one beseechingly in the face, as if in search of some chance consolation, some lost hope; modest young girls returning from long and late labor to a cheerless home, and shrinking more tearfully than indignantly from the glances of ruffians, whose direct contact, even, could not be avoided; women of the town of all kinds and of all ages—the unequivocal beauty in the prime of her womanhood, putting one in mind of the statue in Lucian, with the surface of Parian marble, and the interior filled with filth—the loathsome and utterly lost leper in rags—the wrinkled, bejewelled and paint-begrimed beldame, making a last effort at youth—the mere child of immature form, yet, from long association, an adept in the dreadful coquetries of her trade, and burning with a rabid ambition to be ranked the equal of her elders in vice; drunkards innumerable and inde-scribable—some in shreds and patches, reeling, inarticulate, with bruised vis-age and lack-lustre eyes—some in whole although filthy garments, with a slightly unsteady swagger, thick sensual lips, and hearty-looking rubicund faces—others clothed in materials which had once been good, and which even now were scrupulously well brushed—men who walked with a more than naturally firm and springy step, but whose countenances were fearfully pale, and whose eyes were hideously wild and red, and who clutched with quiver-ing fingers, as they strode through the crowd, at every object which came with-in their reach; beside these, pie-men, porters, coal-heavers, sweeps; organ-grinders, monkey-exhibiters, and ballad mongers, those who vended with those who sang; ragged artizans and exhausted laborers of every description, and all full of a noisy and inordinate vivacity which jarred discordantly upon the ear, and gave an aching sensation to the eye.

As the night deepened, so deepened to me the interest of the scene; for not only did the general character of the crowd materially alter (its gentler features retiring in the gradual withdrawal of the more orderly portion of the people, and its harsher ones coming out into bolder relief, as the late hour brought forth every species of infamy from its den,) but the rays of the gas-lamps, fee-ble at first in their struggle with the dying day, had now at length gained ascendancy, and threw over every thing a fitful and garish lustre. All was dark yet splendid—as that ebony to which has been likened the style of Tertullian.

The wild effects of the light enchained me to an examination of individual faces; and although the rapidity with which the world of light flitted before the window prevented me from casting more than a glance upon each visage, still it seemed that, in my then peculiar mental state, I could frequently read, even in that brief interval of a glance, the history of long years.

With my brow to the glass, I was thus occupied in scrutinizing the mob, when suddenly there came into view a countenance (that of a decrepid old man, some sixty-five or seventy years of age,)—a countenance which at once arrested and absorbed my whole attention, on account of the absolute idiosyncracy of its expression. Any thing even remotely resembling that expression I had never seen before. I well remember that my first thought, upon beholding it, was that Retzch, had he viewed it, would have greatly preferred it to his own pictural incarnations of the fiend. As I endeavored, during the brief minute of my original survey, to form some analysis of the meaning conveyed, there arose confusedly and paradoxically within my mind, the ideas of vast mental power, of caution, of penuriousness, of avarice, of coolness, of malice, of bloodthirstiness, of triumph, of merriment, of excessive terror, of intense—of supreme despair. I felt singularly aroused, startled, fascinated. "How wild a history," I said to myself, "is written within that bosom!" Then came a craving desire to keep the man in view—to know more of him. Hurriedly putting on an overcoat, and seizing my hat and cane, I made my way into the street, and pushed through the crowd in the direction which I had seen him take; for he had already disappeared. With some little difficulty I at length came within sight of him, approached, and followed him closely, yet cautiously, so as not to attract his attention.

I had now a good opportunity of examining his person. He was short in stature, very thin, and apparently very feeble. His clothes, generally, were filthy and ragged; but as he came, now and then, within the strong glare of a lamp, I perceived that his linen, although dirty, was of beautiful texture; and my vision deceived me, or, through a rent in a closely buttoned and evidently second-handed *roquelaure* which enveloped him, I caught a glimpse both of a diamond and of a dagger. These observations heightened my curiosity, and I resolved to follow the stranger whithersoever he should go.

It was now fully night-fall, and a thick humid fog hung over the city, soon ending in a settled and heavy rain. This change of weather had an odd effect upon the crowd, the whole of which was at once put into new commotion, and overshadowed by a world of umbrellas. The waver, the jostle, and the hum increased in a tenfold degree. For my own part I did not much regard the rain—the lurking of an old fever in my system rendering the moisture some-what too dangerously pleasant. Tying a handkerchief about my mouth, I kept on. For half an hour the old man held his way with difficulty along the great thoroughfare; and I here walked close at his elbow through fear of losing sight of him. Never once turning his head to look back, he did not observe me. By and by he passed into a cross street, which, although densely filled with peo-ple, was not quite so much thronged as the main one he had quitted. Here a change in his demeanor became evident. He walked more slowly and with less object than before—more hesitatingly. He crossed and re-crossed the way repeatedly, without apparent aim; and the press was still so thick, that, at every such movement, I was obliged to follow him closely. The street was a narrow and long one, and his course lay within it for nearly an hour, during which the passengers had gradually diminished to about that number which is ordinarily seen at noon in Broadway near the Park—so vast a difference is there between a London populace and that of the most frequented American city. A second turn brought us into a square, brilliantly lighted, and overflowing with life. The old manner of the stranger re-appeared. His chin fell upon his breast, while his eyes rolled wildly from under his knit brows, in every direction, upon those who hemmed him in. He urged his way steadily and perseveringly. I was surprised, however, to find, upon his having made the circuit of the square, that he turned and retraced his steps. Still more was I astonished to see him repeat the same walk several times—once nearly detecting me as he came around with a sudden movement.

In this exercise he spent another hour, at the end of which we met with far less interruption from passengers than at first. The rain fell fast; the air grew cool; and the people were retiring to their homes. With a gesture of impa-tience, the wanderer passed into a bye-street comparatively deserted. Down this, some quarter of a mile long, he rushed with an activity I could not have dreamed of seeing in one so aged, and which put me to much trouble in pur-suit. A few minutes brought us to a large and busy bazaar, with the localities of which the stranger appeared well acquainted, and where his original demeanor again became apparent, as he forced his way to and fro, without aim, among the host of buyers and sellers.

During the hour and a half, or thereabouts, which we passed in this place, it required much caution on my part to keep him within reach without attracting his observation. Luckily I wore a pair of caoutchouc over-shoes, and could move about in perfect silence. At no moment did he see that I watched him. He entered shop after shop, priced nothing, spoke no word, and looked at all objects with a wild and vacant stare. I was now utterly amazed at his behaviour, and firmly resolved that we should not part until I had satisfied myself in some measure respecting him.

A loud-toned clock struck eleven, and the company were fast deserting the bazaar. A shop-keeper, in putting up a shutter, jostled the old man, and at the instant I saw a strong shudder come over his frame. He hurried into the street, looked anxiously around him for an instant, and then ran with incredible swiftness through many crooked and people-less lanes, until we emerged once more upon the great thoroughfare whence we had started—the street of the D— Hotel. It no longer wore, however, the same aspect. It was still brilliant with gas; but the rain fell fiercely, and there were few persons to be seen. The stranger grew pale. He walked moodily some paces up the once populous avenue, then, with a heavy sigh, turned in the direction of the river, and, plunging through a great variety of devious ways, came out, at length, in view of one of the principal theatres. It was about being closed, and the audience were thronging from the doors. I saw the old man gasp as if for breath while he threw himself amid the crowd; but I thought that the intense agony of his countenance had, in some measure, abated. His head again fell upon his breast; he appeared as I had seen him at first. I observed that he now took the course in which had gone the greater number of the audience—but, upon the whole, I was at a loss to comprehend the waywardness of his actions.

As he proceeded, the company grew more scattered, and his old uneasiness and vacillation were resumed. For some time he followed closely a party of some ten or twelve roisterers; but from this number one by one dropped off, until three only remained together, in a narrow and gloomy lane little frequented. The stranger paused, and, for a moment, seemed lost in thought; then, with every mark of agitation, pursued rapidly a route which brought us to the verge of the city, amid regions very different from those we had hitherto traversed. It was the most noisome quarter of London, where every thing wore the worst impress of the most deplorable poverty, and of the most desperate crime. By the dim light of an accidental lamp, tall, antique, worm-eaten, wooden tenements were seen tottering to their fall, in directions so many and capricious that scarce the semblance of a passage was discernible between them. The paving-stones lay at random, displaced from their beds by the rankly-growing grass. Horrible filth festered in the dammed-up gutters. The whole atmosphere teemed with desolation. Yet, as we proceeded, the sounds of human life revived by sure degrees, and at length large bands of the most abandoned of a London populace were seen reeling to and fro. The spirits of the old man again flickered up, as a lamp which is near its death-hour. Once more he strode onward with elastic tread. Suddenly a corner was turned, a blaze of light burst upon our sight, and we stood before one of the huge suburban temples of Intemperance—one of the palaces of the fiend, Gin.

It was now nearly day-break; but a number of wretched inebriates still pressed in and out of the flaunting entrance. With a half shriek of joy the old man forced a passage within, resumed at once his original bearing, and stalked backward and forward, without apparent object, among the throng. He had not been thus long occupied, however, before a rush to the doors gave token that the host was closing them for the night. It was something even more intense than despair that I then observed upon the countenance of the singular being whom I had watched so pertinaciously. Yet he did not hesitate in his career, but, with a mad energy, retraced his steps at once, to the heart of the mighty London. Long and swiftly he fled, while I followed him in the wildest amazement, resolute not to abandon a scrutiny in which I now felt an interest all-absorbing. The sun arose while we proceeded, and, when we had once again reached that most thronged mart of the populous town, the street of the D— Hotel, it presented an appearance of human bustle and activity scarcely inferior to what I had seen on the evening before. And here, long, amid the momently increasing confusion, did I persist in my pursuit of the stranger. But, as usual, he walked to and fro, and during the day did not pass from out the turmoil of that street. And, as the shades of the second evening came on, I grew wearied unto death, and, stopping fully in front of the wanderer, gazed at him steadfastly in the face. He noticed me not, but resumed his solemn walk, while I, ceasing to follow, remained absorbed in contemplation. "This old man," I said at length, "is the type and the genius of deep crime. He refuses to be alone. *He is the man of the crowd*. It will be in vain to follow, for I shall learn no more of him, nor of his deeds. The worst heart of the world is a grosser book than the 'Hortulus Animae,'* and perhaps it is but one of the great mercies of God that *"er lasst sich nicht lesen."*

* The *"Hortulus Animae cum Oratiunculis Aliquibus Superadditis"* of Grünninger.

Charles Dickens
FROM MARTIN CHUZZLEWIT

Mr Pecksniff's horse being regarded in the light of a sacred animal, only to be driven by him, the chief priest of that temple, or by some person distinctly nominated for the time being to that high office by himself, the two young men agreed to walk to Salisbury; and so, when the time came, they set off on foot; which was, after all, a better mode of travelling than in the gig, as the weather was very cold and very dry.

Better! A rare strong, hearty, healthy walk—four statute miles an hour—preferable to that rumbling, tumbling, jolting, shaking, scraping, creaking, villainous old gig? Why, the two things will not admit of comparison. It is an insult to the walk, to set them side by side. Where is an instance of a gig having ever circulated a man's blood, unless when, putting him in danger of his neck, it awakened in his veins and in his ears, and all along his spine, a tingling heat, much more peculiar than agreeable? When did a gig ever sharpen anybody's wits and energies, unless it was when the horse bolted, and, crashing madly down a steep hill with a stone wall at the bottom, his desperate circumstances suggested to the only gentleman left inside, some novel and unheard-of mode of dropping out behind? Better than the gig!

The air was cold, Tom; so it was, there was no denying it; but would it have been more genial in the gig? The blacksmith's fire burned very bright, and leaped up high, as though it wanted men to warm; but would it have been less tempting, looked at from the clammy cushions of a gig? The wind blew keenly, nipping the features of the hardy wight who fought his way along; blinding him with his own hair if he had enough of it, and wintry dust if he hadn't; stopping his breath as though he had been soused in a cold bath; tearing aside his wrappings-up, and whistling in the very marrow of his bones; but it would have done all this a hundred times more fiercely to a man in a gig, wouldn't it? A fig for gigs!

Better than the gig! When were travellers by wheels and hoofs seen with

such red-hot cheeks as those? when were they so good-humouredly and merrily bloused? when did their laughter ring upon the air, as they turned them
round, what time the stronger gusts came sweeping up; and, facing round
again as they passed by, dashed on, in such a glow of ruddy health as nothing
could keep pace with, but the high spirits it engendered? Better than the gig!
Why, here *is* a man in a gig coming the same way now. Look at him as he
passes his whip into his left hand, chafes his numbed right fingers on his granite leg, and beats those marble toes of his upon the foot-board. Ha, ha, ha!
Who would exchange this rapid hurry of the blood for yonder stagnant misery,
though its pace were twenty miles for one?

Better than the gig! No man in a gig could have such interest in the milestones. No man in a gig could see, or feel, or think, like merry users of their
legs. How, as the wind sweeps on, upon these breezy downs, it tracks its flight
in darkening ripples on the grass, and smoothest shadows on the hills! Look
round and round upon this bare bleak plain, and see even here, upon a winter's day, how beautiful the shadows are! Alas! it is the nature of their kind to
be so. The loveliest things in life, Tom, are but shadows; and they come and
go, and change and fade away, as rapidly as these!

John Clare
THE MORES

Far spread the moorey ground a level scene
Bespread with rush and one eternal green
That never felt the rage of blundering plough
Though centurys wreathed springs blossoms on its brow
Still meeting plains that stretched them far away
In uncheckt shadows of green brown and grey
Unbounded freedom ruled the wandering scene
Nor fence of ownership crept in between
To hide the prospect of the following eye
Its only bondage was the circling sky
One mighty flat undwarfed by bush and tree
Spread its faint shadow of immensity
And lost itself which seemed to eke its bounds
In the blue mist the orisons edge surrounds
Now this sweet vision of my boyish hours
Free as spring clouds and wild as summer flowers
Is faded all—a hope that blossomed free
And hath been once no more shall ever be
Inclosure came and trampled on the grave
Of labours rights and left the poor a slave
And memorys pride ere want to wealth did bow
Is both the shadow and the substance now
The sheep and cows were free to range as then
Where change might prompt nor felt the bonds of men
Cows went and came with evening morn and night
To the wild pasture as their common right
And sheep unfolded with the rising sun
Heard the swains shout and felt their freedom won

Tracked the red fallow field and heath and plain
Then met the brook and drank and roamed again
The brook that dribbled on as clear as glass
Beneath the roots they hid among the grass
While the glad shepherd traced their tracks along
Free as the lark and happy as her song
But now alls fled and flats of many a dye
That seemed to lengthen with the following eye
Moors loosing from the sight far smooth and blea
Where swept the plover in its pleasure free
Are vanished now with commons wild and gay
As poets visions of lifes early day
Mulberry bushes where the boy would run
To fill his hands with fruit are grubbed and done
And hedgrow briars—flower lovers overjoyed
Came and got flower pots—these are all destroyed
And sky bound mores in mangled garbs are left
Like mighty giants of their limbs bereft
Fence now meets fence in owners little bounds
Of field and meadow large as garden grounds
In little parcels little minds to please
With men and flocks imprisoned ill at ease
Each little path that led its pleasant way
As sweet as morning leading night astray
Where little flowers bloomed round a varied host
That travel felt delighted to be lost
Nor grudged the steps that he had taen as vain
When right roads traced his journeys end again
Nay on a broken tree hed sit awhile
To see the mores and fields and meadows smile
Sometimes with cowslaps smothered—then all white
With daiseys—then the summers splendid sight
Of corn fields crimson oer the 'headach' bloomd
Like splendid armys for the battle plumed
He gazed upon them with wild fancys eye

As fallen landscapes from an evening sky
These paths are stopt—the rude philistines thrall
Is laid upon them and destroyed them all
Each little tyrant with his little sign
Shows where man claims earth glows no more divine
On paths to freedom and to childhood dear
A board sticks up to notice 'no road here'
And on the tree with ivy overhung
The hated sign by vulgar taste is hung
As tho the very birds should learn to know
When they go there they must no further go
This with the poor scared freedom bade good bye
And much they feel it in the smothered sigh
And birds and trees and flowers without a name
All sighed when lawless laws enclosure came
And dreams of plunder in such rebel schemes
Have found too truly that they were but dreams

Southern Paiute
A MORNING WALK

Over the land over the land
I walked at morn
Singing and trembling with cold

Matsuo Bashō

FROM THE NARROW ROAD TO THE INTERIOR

Translated by Sam Hamill

The moon and sun are eternal travelers. Even the years wander on. A lifetime adrift in a boat, or in old age leading a tired horse into the years, every day is a journey, and the journey itself is home. From the earliest times there have always been some who perished along the road. Still I have always been drawn by windblown clouds into dreams of a lifetime of wandering. Coming home from a year's walking tour of the coast last autumn, I swept the cobwebs from my hut on the banks of the Sumida just in time for New Year, but by the time spring mists began to rise from the fields, I longed to cross the Shirakawa Barrier into the Northern Interior. Drawn by the wanderer-spirit Dōsojin, I couldn't concentrate on things. Mending my cotton pants, sewing a new strap on my bamboo hat, I daydreamed. Rubbing moxa into my legs to strengthen them, I dreamed a bright moon rising over Matsushima. So I placed my house in another's hands and moved to my patron Mr. Sampū's summer house in preparation for my journey. And I left a verse by my door:

Even this grass hut
may be transformed
into a doll's house

Very early on the twenty-seventh morning of the third moon, under a predawn haze, transparent moon still visible, Mount Fuji just a shadow, I set out under the cherry blossoms of Ueno and Yanaka. When would I see them again? A few old friends had gathered in the night and followed along far enough to see me off from the boat. Getting off at Senju, I felt three thousand miles rushing through my heart, the whole world only a dream. I saw it through farewell tears.

Spring passes
and the birds cry out—
tears in the eyes of fishes

With these first words from my brush, I started. Those who remain behind
watch the shadow of a traveler's back disappear.

The second year of Genroku [1689], I think of the long way leading into
the Northern Interior under Go stone skies. My hair may turn white as frost
before I return from those fabled places—or maybe I won't return at all. By
nightfall, we come to Sōka, bony shoulders sore from heavy pack, grateful for
warm night robe, cotton bathing gown, writing brush, ink stone, necessities..
The pack made heavier by farewell gifts from friends. I couldn't leave them
behind.

Once in Kurobane, I visited the powerful samurai Jōbōji, overseer of the
manor. Surprised by the visit, he kept me up talking through several days and
nights, often at the home of his brother Tōsui. We visited their relatives and
friends. One day we walked out to Inu oumono, Dog-shooting Grounds. We
walked out into the moors to find the tomb of Lady Tamamo, who turned herself to stone. We paid homage at Hachiman Shrine, where Yoshitsune's general Yoichi shot a fan from a passing boat after praying to Shō-hachiman, war-
rior-god of this shrine. At dusk we returned to Tōsui's home.
    Invited to visit Shūgen Kōmyō Temple's hall for mountain monks:

In summer mountains
bow to holy high water clogs
bless this long journey

In a mountain hermitage near Ungan Temple, my dharma master Butcho
wrote:

A five-foot thatched hut:
I wouldn't even put it up
but for the failing rain

He inscribed the poem on a rock with charcoal—he told me long ago. Curious, several young people joined in, walking sticks pointed toward Ungan Temple. We were so caught up in talking we arrived at the temple unexpectedly. Through the long valley, under dense cedar and pine with dripping moss, below a cold spring sky—through the viewing gardens, we crossed a bridge and entered the temple gate.

I searched out back for Butchō's hermitage and found it up the hill, near a cave on a rocky ridge—like the cave where Myōzenji lived for fifteen years, like Zen master Houn's retreat.

> Even woodpeckers leave it alone:
> a hermitage
> in a summer grove

One small poem, quickly written, pinned to a post.

We crossed over the Natorigawa on the seventh day, fifth moon, and entered Sendai on the day we tie blue iris to the eaves and pray for health. We found an inn and decided to spend several days. I'd heard of a painter here, Kaemon, who was a kindred spirit and had visited all the nearby places the poets had made famous. Before him, these places were all but forgotten. He agreed to be our guide. The fields at Miyagi were carpeted with bush clover that would bloom in autumn. In Tamada and Yokono and at Azalea Hill there were andromeda flowers in bloom. Passing through pine woods sunlight couldn't penetrate, we came to Kinoshita, the "Under Woods" where the poet in the *Kokinshū* begged an umbrella for his lord in falling dew. We visited Yakushido Shrine and the Shrine of Tenjin until the sun went down. Later the painter gave us drawings of Matsushima and Shiogama. And two pairs of new straw sandals with iris-blue straps—*hanamuke,* farewell gifts. He was a truly kindred spirit.

> To have blue irises
> blooming on one's feet:
> walking-sandal straps

Checking Kaemon's drawings as we walked, we followed the *oku-no-hosomichi* along the mountainside where sedge grass grew tall in bunches. The Tofu area is famous for its sedge mats, sent in tribute to the governor each year.

At Taga Castle we found the most ancient monument Tsubo-no-ishibumi, in Ichikawa Village. It's about six feet high and three feet wide. We struggled to read the inscription under heavy moss:

THIS CASTLE WAS BUILT BY SHOGUN ONO-NO-AZUMABITO IN 724. IN 762, HIS MAJESTY'S COMMANDING GENERAL, EMI-NO-ASAKARI, SUPERVISED REPAIRS.

Dated from the time of Emperor Shōmu, Tsubo-no-ishibumi inspired many a poet. Floods and landslides buried trails and markers, trees have grown and died, making this monument very difficult to find. The past remains hidden in clouds of memory. Still it returned us to memories from a thousand years before. Such a moment is the reason for a pilgrimage: infirmities forgotten, the ancients remembered, joyous tears trembled in my eyes.

We stopped along the Tama River at Noda, and at the huge stone in the lake, Oki-no-ishi, both made famous in poems. On Mount Sue-no-matsu, we found a temple called Masshozan. There were graves everywhere among the pines, underscoring Po Chu-i's famous lines quoted in *The Tale of Genji,* "wing and wing, branch and branch," and I thought, "Yes, what we all must come to," my sadness heavy.

At Shiogama Beach, a bell sounded evening. The summer rain-sky cleared to reveal a pale moon high over Magaki Island. I remembered the "fishing boats pulling together" in a *Kokinshū* poem, and understood it clearly for the first time.

Along the Michinoku
every place is wonderful,
but in Shiogama
fishing boats pulling together
are most amazing of all

That night we were entertained by a blind singer playing a lute to boisterous back-country ballads one hears only deep inside the country, not like the songs in *The Tale of the Heike* or the dance songs. A real earful, but pleased to hear the tradition continued.

Rose at dawn to pay respects at Myōjin Shrine in Shiogama. The former governor rebuilt it with huge, stately pillars, bright-painted rafters, and a long stone walkway rising steeply under a morning sun that danced and flashed along the red lacquered fence. I thought, "As long as the road is, even if it ends in dust, the gods come with us, keeping a watchful eye. This is our culture's greatest gift." Kneeling at the shrine, I noticed a fine old lantern with this inscribed on its iron grate:

IN THE THIRD YEAR OF THE BUNJI ERA [1187]

DEDICATED BY IZUMI SABURŌ

Suddenly, five long centuries passed before my eyes. A trusted, loyal man martyred by his brother; today there's not a man alive who doesn't revere his name. As he himself would say, a man must follow the Confucian model— renown will inevitably result.

Early morning of the twelfth day, fifth moon. We started out for Hiraizumi, intending to go by way of the famous Aneha Pine and the Odae Bridge. The trail was narrow and little-traveled—only the occasional woodcutter or hunter. We took a wrong road and ended up in the port town of Ishinomaki on a broad bay with Mount Kinka in the distance. Yakamochi has a poem for the emperor in the *Man'yōshū* saying Kinka's "where gold blossoms." It rises across water cluttered with cargo boats and fishing boats, shoreline packed with houses, smoke rising from their stoves. Our unplanned visit prompted an immediate search for lodging. No one made an offer. Spent the night in a cold shack and left again at daybreak, following unknown paths. We passed near the Sode Ferry, Obuchi Meadow, and the Mano Moor—all made famous in poems. After crossing a long miserable marsh, we stayed at Toima, pushing on to Hiraizumi in the morning. An arduous trek of over forty difficult miles in two days.

Here three generations of the Fujiwara clan passed as though in a dream. The great outer gates lay in ruins. Where Hidehira's manor stood, rice fields grew. Only Mount Kinkei remained. I climbed the hill where Yoshitsune died; I saw the Kitakami, a broad stream flowing down through the Nambu Plain, the Koromo River circling Izumi Castle below the hill before joining the Kitakami. The ancient ruins of Yasuhira—from the end of the Golden Era—lie out beyond the Koromo Barrier where they stood guard against the Ainu people. The faithful elite remained bound to the castle, for all their valor, reduced to ordinary grass. Tu Fu wrote:

> The whole country devastated,
> only mountains and rivers remain.
> In springtime, at the ruined castle,
> the grass is always green.

We sat awhile, our hats for a seat, seeing it all through tears.

> Summer grasses:
> all that remains of great soldiers'
> imperial dreams

Sora wrote:

> Kanefusa's
> own white hair
> seen in blossoming briar

Two temple halls I longed to see were finally opened at Chuson Temple. In the Sutra Library, Kyōdō, statues of the three generals of Hiraizumi; and in the Hall of Light, Hikaridō, their coffins and images of three buddhas. It would have all fallen down, jeweled doors battered by winds, gold pillars cracked by cold, all would have gone to grass, but added outer roof and walls protect it. Through the endless winds and rains of a thousand years, this great hall remains.

> Fifth-month rains hammer
> and blow but never quite touch
> Hikaridō

The road through the Nambu Plain visible in the distance, we stayed the night in Iwate, then trudged on past Cape Oguro and Mizu Island, both along the river. Beyond Narugo Hot Springs, we crossed Shitomae Barrier and entered Dewa Province. Almost no one comes this way, and the barrier guards were suspicious, slow, and thorough. Delayed, we climbed a steep mountain in falling dark and took refuge in a guard shack. A heavy storm pounded the shack with wind and rain for three miserable days.

Eaten alive by lice and fleas
now the horse
beside my pillow pees

The guard told us, "To get to Dewa, you'd better take a guide. There's a high mountain and a hard-to-find trail." He found us a powerful young man, short sword on his hip and oak walking stick in hand, and off we went, not without a little trepidation. As forewarned, the mountain was steep, the trail narrow, not even a birdcall to be heard. We made our way through deep forest dark as night, reminding me of Tu Fu's poem about "clouds bringing darkness." We groped through thick bamboo, waded streams, climbed through rocks, sweaty, fearful, and tired, until we finally came to the village of Mogami. Our guide, turning back, said again how the trail was tough. "Happy you didn't meet many surprises!" And departed. Hearing this, our hearts skipped another beat.

Today we came through places with names like Children-Desert-Parents, Lost Children, Send-Back-the-Dog, and Turn-Back-the-Horse—some of the most fearsomely dangerous places in all the North Country. And well named. Weakened and exhausted, I went to bed early but was roused by the voices of two young women in the room next door. Then an old man's voice joined theirs. They were prostitutes from Niigata in Echigo Province and were on their way to Ise Shrine in the south, the old man seeing them off at this barrier, Ichiburi. He would turn back to Niigata in the morning, carrying their letters home. One girl quoted the *Shinkokinshū* poem, "On the beach where white waves fall, / we all wander like children into every circumstance, / carried forward every day. . . ." And as they bemoaned their fate in life, I fell asleep.

In the morning, preparing to leave, they came to ask directions. "May we follow along behind?" they asked. "We're lost and not a little fearful. Your robes bring the spirit of the Buddha to our journey." They had mistaken us for priests. "Our way includes detours and retreats," I told them. "But follow anyone on this road, and the gods will see you through." I hated to leave them in tears and thought about them hard for a long time after we left. I told Sora, and he wrote down:

Under one roof, prostitute and priest,
we all sleep together:
moon in a field of clover

Charles Dickens
NIGHT WALKS

Some years ago, a temporary inability to sleep, referable to a distressing impression, caused me to walk about the streets all night, for a series of several nights. The disorder might have taken a long time to conquer, if it had been faintly experimented on in bed; but, it was soon defeated by the brisk treatment of getting up directly after lying down, and going out, and coming home tired at sunrise.

In the course of those nights, I finished my education in a fair amateur experience of houselessness. My principal object being to get through the night, the pursuit of it brought me into sympathetic relations with people who have no other object every night in the year.

The month was March, and the weather damp, cloudy, and cold. The sun not rising before half-past five, the night perspective looked sufficiently long at half-past twelve: which was about my time for confronting it.

The restlessness of a great city, and the way in which it tumbles and tosses before it can get to sleep, formed one of the first entertainments offered to the contemplation of us houseless people. It lasted about two hours. We lost a great deal of companionship when the late public-houses turned their lamps out, and when the potmen thrust the last brawling drunkards into the street; but stray vehicles and stray people were left us, after that. If we were very lucky, a policeman's rattle sprang and a fray turned up; but, in general, surprisingly little of this diversion was provided. Except in the Haymarket, which is the worst kept part of London, and about Kent-street in the Borough, and along a portion of the line of the Old Kent-road, the peace was seldom violently broken. But, it was always the case that London, as if in imitation of individual citizens belonging to it, had expiring fits and starts of restlessness. After all seemed quiet, if one cab rattled by, half-a-dozen would surely follow; and Houselessness even observed that intoxicated people appeared to be magnetically attracted towards each other: so that we knew when we saw one drunken object staggering against the shutters of a shop, that another drunken object would stagger up before five minutes were out, to fraternise or fight with it. When we made a divergence from the regular species of drunkard, the thin-armed, puff-faced, leaden-lipped gin-drinker, and encountered a rarer specimen of a more decent appearance, fifty to one but that specimen was dressed in soiled mourning. As the street experience in the night, so the street experience in the day; the common folk who come unexpectedly into a little property, come unexpectedly into a deal of liquor.

At length these flickering sparks would die away, worn out—the last veritable sparks of waking life trailed from some late pieman or hot-potato man—and London would sink to rest. And then the yearning of the houseless mind would be for any sign of company, any lighted place, any movement, anything suggestive of any one being up—nay, even so much as awake, for the houseless eye looked out for lights in windows.

Walking the streets under the pattering rain, Houselessness would walk and walk and walk, seeing nothing but the interminable tangle of streets, save at a corner, here and there, two policemen in conversation, or the sergeant or inspector looking after his men. Now and then in the night—but rarely—Houselessness would become aware of a furtive head peering out of a doorway a few yards before him, and, coming up with the head, would find a man standing bolt upright to keep within the doorway's shadow, and evidently intent upon no particular service to society. Under a kind of fascination, and in a ghostly silence suitable to the time, Houselessness and this gentleman would eye one another from head to foot, and so, without exchange of speech, part, mutually suspicious. Drip, drip, drip, from ledge and coping, splash from pipes and water-spouts, and by-and-by the houseless shadow would fall upon the stones that pave the way to Waterloo-bridge; it being in the houseless mind to have a halfpenny worth of excuse for saying "Good night" to the toll-keeper, and catching a glimpse of his fire. A good fire and a good great-coat and a good woollen neck-shawl, were comfortable things to see in conjunction with the toll-keeper; also his brisk wakefulness was excellent company when he rattled the change of halfpence down upon that metal table of his, like a man who defied the night, with all its sorrowful thoughts, and didn't care for the coming of dawn. There was need of encouragement on the threshold of the bridge, for the bridge was dreary. The chopped-up murdered man, had not been lowered with a rope over the parapet when those nights were; he was alive, and slept then quietly enough most likely, and undisturbed by any dream of where he was to come. But the river had an awful look, the buildings on the banks were muffled in black shrouds, and the reflected lights seemed to originate deep in the water, as if the spectres of suicides were holding them to show where they went down. The wild moon and clouds were as restless as an evil conscience in a tumbled bed, and the very shadow of the immensity of London seemed to lie oppressively upon the river.

Between the bridge and the two great theatres, there was but the distance of a few hundred paces, so the theatres came next. Grim and black within, at night, those great dry Wells, and lonesome to imagine, with the rows of faces faded out, the lights extinguished, and the seats all empty, one would think that nothing in them knew itself at such a time but Yorick's skull. In one of my night walks, as the church steeples were shaking the March winds and rain with strokes of Four, I passed the outer boundary of one of these great deserts, and entered it. With a dim lantern in my hand, I groped my well-known way to the stage and looked over the orchestra—which was like a great grave dug for a time of pestilence—into the void beyond. A dismal cavern of an immense aspect, with the chandelier gone dead like everything else, and nothing visible through mist and fog and space, but tiers of winding-sheets. The ground at my feet where, when last there, I had seen the peasantry of Naples dancing among the vines, reckless of the burning mountain which threatened to overwhelm them, was now in possession of a strong serpent of engine-hose, watchfully lying in wait for the serpent Fire, and ready to fly at it if it showed its forked tongue. A ghost of a watchman, carrying a faint corpse candle, haunted the distant upper gallery and flitted away. Retiring within the proscenium, and holding my light above my head towards the rolled-up curtain—green no more, but black as ebony—my sight lost itself in a gloomy vault, showing faint indications in it of a shipwreck of canvas and cordage. Methought I felt much as a diver might, at the bottom of the sea.

In those small hours when there was no movement in the streets, it afforded matter for reflection to take Newgate in the way, and, touching its rough stone, to think of the prisoners in their sleep, and then to glance in at the lodge over the spiked wicket, and see the fire and light of the watching turnkeys, on the white wall. Not an inappropriate time either, to linger by that wicked little

Debtors' Door—shutting tighter than any other door one ever saw—which has been Death's Door to so many. In the days of the uttering of forged one-pound notes by people tempted up from the country, how many hundreds of wretched creatures of both sexes—many quite innocent—swung out of a piti-less and inconsistent world, with the tower of yonder Christian church of Saint Sepulchre monstrously before their eyes! Is there any haunting of the Bank Parlour, by the remorseful souls of old directors, in the nights of these later days, I wonder, or is it as quiet as this degenerate Aceldama of an Old Bailey?

To walk on to the Bank, lamenting the good old times and bemoaning the present evil period, would be an easy next step, so I would take it, and would make my houseless circuit of the Bank, and give a thought to the treasure within; likewise to the guard of soldiers passing the night there, and nodding over the fire. Next, I went to Billingsgate, in some hope of market-people, but it proving as yet too early, crossed London-bridge and got down by the water-side on the Surrey shore among the buildings of the great brewery. There was plenty going on at the brewery; and the reek, and the smell of grains, and the rattling of the plump dray horses at their mangers, were capital company. Quite refreshed by having mingled with this good society, I made a new start with a new heart, setting the old King's Bench prison before me for my next object, and resolving, when I should come to the wall, to think of poor Horace Kinch, and the Dry Rot in men.

A very curious disease the Dry Rot in men, and difficult to detect the beginning of. It had carried Horace Kinch inside the wall of the old King's Bench prison, and it had carried him out with his feet foremost. He was a like-ly man to look at, in the prime of life, well to do, as clever as he needed to be, and popular among many friends. He was suitably married, and had healthy and pretty children. But, like some fair-looking houses or fair-looking ships, he took the Dry Rot. The first strong external revelation of the Dry Rot in men is a tendency to lurk and lounge; to be at street-comers without intelligible rea-son; to be going anywhere when met; to be about many places rather than at any; to do nothing tangible, but to have an intention of performing a variety of intangible duties to-morrow or the day after. When this manifestation of the disease is observed, the observer will usually connect it with a vague impres-sion once formed or received, that the patient was living a little too hard. He will scarcely have had leisure to turn it over in his mind and form the terrible suspicion "Dry Rot," when he will notice a change for the worse in the patient's appearance: a certain slovenliness and deterioration, which is not poverty, nor dirt, nor intoxication, nor ill-health, but simply Dry Rot. To this, succeeds a smell as of strong waters, in the morning; to that, a looseness respecting money; to that, a stronger smell as of strong waters, at all times; to that, a looseness respecting everything; to that, a trembling of the limbs, somnolency, misery, and crumbling to pieces. As it is in wood, so it is in men. Dry Rot advances at a compound usury quite incalculable. A plank is found infected with it, and the whole structure is devoted. Thus it had been with the unhappy Horace Kinch, lately buried by a small subscription. Those who knew him had not nigh done saying, "So well off, so comfortably established, with such hope before him—and yet, it is feared, with a slight touch of Dry Rot!" when lo! the man was all Dry Rot and dust.

From the dead wall associated on those houseless nights with this too common story, I chose next to wander by Bethlehem Hospital; partly, because it lay on my road round to Westminster; partly, because I had a night fancy in my head which could be best pursued within sight of its walls and dome. And the fancy was this: Are not the sane and the insane equal at night as the sane lie a dreaming? Are not all of us outside this hospital, who dream, more or less in the condition of those inside it, every night of our lives? Are we not nightly persuaded, as they daily are, that we associate preposterously with kings and queens, emperors and empresses, and notabilities of all sorts? Do we not nightly jumble events and personages and times and places, as these do daily? Are we not sometimes troubled by our own sleeping inconsistencies, and do we not vexedly try to account for them or excuse them, just as these do sometimes in respect of their waking delusions? Said an afflicted man to me, when I was last in a hospital like this, "Sir, I can frequently fly." I was half ashamed to reflect that so could I—by night. Said a woman to me on the same occasion, "Queen Victoria frequently comes to dine with me, and her Majesty and I dine off peaches and maccaroni in our night-gowns, and his Royal Highness the Prince Consort does us the honour to make a third on horseback in a Field-Marshal's uniform." Could I refrain from reddening with consciousness when I remembered the amazing royal parties I myself had given (at night), the unaccountable viands I had put on table, and my extraordinary manner of conducting myself on those distinguished occasions? I wonder that the great master who knew everything, when he called Sleep the death of each day's life, did not call Dreams the insanity of each day's sanity.

By this time I had left the Hospital behind me, and was again setting towards the river; and in a short breathing space I was on Westminster-bridge, regaling my houseless eyes with the external walls of the British Parliament—the perfection of a stupendous institution, I know, and the admiration of all surrounding nations and succeeding ages, I do not doubt, but perhaps a little the better now and then for being pricked up to its work. Turning off into Old Palace-yard, the Courts of Law kept me company for a quarter of an hour; hinting in low whispers what numbers of people they were keeping awake, and how intensely wretched and horrible they were rendering the small hours to unfortunate suitors. Westminster Abbey was fine gloomy society for another quarter of an hour; suggesting a wonderful procession of its dead among the dark arches and pillars, each century more amazed by the century following it than by all the centuries going before. And indeed in those houseless night walks—which even included cemeteries where watchmen went round among the graves at stated times, and moved the tell-tale handle of an index which recorded that they had touched it at such an hour—it was a solemn consideration what enormous hosts of dead belong to one old great city, and how, if they were raised while the living slept, there would not be the space of a pin's point in all the streets and ways for the living to come out into. Not only that, but the vast armies of dead would overflow the hills and valleys beyond the city, and would stretch away all round, it God knows how far.

When a church clock strikes, on houseless ears in the dead of the night, it may be at first mistaken for company and hailed as such. But, as the spreading circles of vibration, which you may perceive at such a time with great clearness, go opening out, for ever and ever afterwards widening perhaps (as the philosopher has suggested) in eternal space, the mistake is rectified and the sense of loneliness is profounder. Once—it was after leaving the Abbey and turning my face north—I came to the great steps of St. Martin's church as the clock was striking Three. Suddenly, a thing that in a moment more I should have trodden upon without seeing, rose up at my feet with a cry of loneliness and houselessness, struck out of it by the bell, the like of which I never heard. We then stood face to face looking at one another, frightened by one another. The creature was like a beetle-browed hair-lipped youth of twenty, and it had a loose bundle of rags on, which it held together with one of its hands. It shivered from head to foot, and its teeth chattered, and as it stared at me—persecutory devil, ghost, whatever it thought me—it made with its whining mouth as if it were snapping at me, like a worried dog. Intending to give this ugly object money, I put out my hand to stay it—for it recoiled as it whined and snapped—and laid my hand upon its shoulder. Instantly, it twisted out of its garment, like the young man in the New Testament, and left me standing alone with its rags in my hands.

Covent-garden Market, when it was market morning, was wonderful company. The great waggons of cabbages, with growers' men and boys lying asleep under them, and with sharp dogs from market-garden neighbourhoods looking after the whole, were as good as a party. But one of the worst night sights I know in London, is to be found in the children who prowl about this place; who sleep in the baskets, fight for the offal, dart at any object they think they can lay their thieving hands on, dive under the carts and barrows, dodge the constables, and are perpetually making a blunt pattering on the pavement of the Piazza with the rain of their naked feet. A painful and unnatural result comes of the comparison one is forced to institute between the growth of corruption as displayed in the so much improved and cared for fruits of the earth, and the growth of corruption as displayed in these all uncared for (except inasmuch as ever-hunted) savages.

There was early coffee to be got about Covent-garden Market, and that was more company—warm company, too, which was better. Toast of a very substantial quality, was likewise procurable: though the towzled-headed man who made it, in an inner chamber within the coffee-room, hadn't got his coat on yet, and was so heavy with sleep that in every interval of toast and coffee he went off anew behind the partition into complicated cross-roads of choke and snore, and lost his way directly. Into one of these establishments (among the earliest) near Bow-street, there came one morning as I sat over my houseless cup, pondering where to go next, a man in a high and long snuff-coloured coat, and shoes, and, to the best of my belief, nothing else but a hat, who took out of his hat a large cold meat pudding; a meat pudding so large that it was a very tight fit, and brought the lining of the hat out with it. This mysterious man was known by his pudding, for on his entering, the man of sleep brought him a pint of hot tea, a small loaf, and a large knife and fork and plate. Left to himself in his box, he stood the pudding on the bare table, and, instead of cutting it, stabbed it, overhand, with the knife, like a mortal enemy; then took the knife out, wiped it on his sleeve, tore the pudding asunder with his fingers, and ate it all up. The remembrance of this man with the pudding remains with me as the remembrance of the most spectral person my houselessness encountered. Twice only was I in that establishment, and twice I saw him stalk in (as I should say, just out of bed, and presently going back to bed), take out his pudding, stab his pudding, wipe the dagger, and eat his pudding all up. He was a man whose figure promised cadaverousness, but who had an excessively red face, though shaped like a horse's. On the second occasion of my seeing him, he said huskily to the man of sleep, "Am I red to-night?" "You are," he uncompromisingly answered. "My mother," said the spectre, "was a red-faced woman that liked drink, and I looked at her hard when she laid in her coffin, and I took the complexion." Somehow, the pudding seemed an unwholesome pudding after that, and I put myself in its way no more.

When there was no market, or when I wanted variety, a railway terminus with the morning mails coming in, was remunerative company. But like most of the company to be had in this world, it lasted only a very short time. The station lamps would burst out ablaze, the porters would emerge from places of concealment, the cabs and trucks would rattle to their places (the post-office carts were already in theirs), and, finally, the bell would strike up, and the train would come banging in. But there were few passengers and little luggage, and everything scuttled away with the greatest expedition. The locomotive post-offices, with their great nets—as if they had been dragging the country for bodies—would fly open as to their doors, and would disgorge a smell of lamp, an exhausted clerk, a guard in a red coat, and their bags of letters; the engine would blow and heave and perspire, like an engine wiping its forehead and saying what a run it had had; and within ten minutes the lamps were out, and I was houseless and alone again.

But now, there were driven cattle on the high road near, wanting (as cattle always do) to turn into the midst of stone walls, and squeeze themselves through six inches' width of iron railing, and getting their heads down (also as cattle always do) for tossing-purchase at quite imaginary dogs, and giving themselves and every devoted creature associated with them a most extraordinary amount of unnecessary trouble. Now, too, the conscious gas began to grow pale with the knowledge that daylight was coming, and straggling work-people were already in the streets, and, as waking life had become extinguished with the last pieman's sparks, so it began to be rekindled with the fires of the first street-corner breakfast-sellers. And so by faster and faster degrees, until the last degrees were very fast, the day came, and I was tired and could sleep. And it is not, as I used to think, going home at such times, the least wonderful thing in London, that in the real desert region of the night, the houseless wanderer is alone there. I knew well enough where to find Vice and Misfortune of all kinds, if I had chosen; but they were put out of sight, and my houselessness had many miles upon miles of streets in which it could, and did, have its own solitary way.

Anne Finch
A NOCTURNAL REVERIE

In such a Night, when every louder Wind
Is to its distant Cavern safe confin'd;
And only gentle Zephyr fans his Wings,
And lonely Philomel, still waking, sings;
Or from some Tree, fam'd for the Owl's delight,
She, hollowing clear, directs the Wand'rer right:
In such a Night, when passing Clouds give place,
Or thinly veil the Heav'ns mysterious Face;
When in some River, overhung with Green,
The waving Moon and trembling Leaves are seen;
When freshen'd Grass now bears itself upright,
And makes cool Banks to pleasing Rest invite,
Whence springs the Woodbind, and the Bramble-Rose,
And where the sleepy Cowslip shelter'd grows;
Whilst now a paler Hue the Foxglove takes,
Yet checquers still with Red the dusky brakes:
When scatter'd Glow-worms, but in Twilight fine,
Shew trivial Beauties, watch their Hour to shine;
Whilst Salisb'ry stands the Test of every Light,
In perfect Charms, and perfect Virtue bright:
When Odours, which declin'd repelling Day,
Thro' temp'rate Air uninterrupted stray;
When darken'd Groves their softest Shadows wear,
And falling Waters we distinctly hear;
When thro' the Gloom more venerable shows
Some ancient Fabrick, awful in Repose,
While Sunburnt Hills their swarthy Looks conceal,
And swelling Haycocks thicken up the Vale:

When the loos'd Horse now, as his Pasture leads,
Comes slowly grazing thro' th' adjoining Meads,
Whose stealing Pace, and lengthen'd Shade we fear,
Till torn-up Forage in his Teeth we hear:
When nibbling Sheep at large pursue their Food,
And unmolested Kine rechew the Cud;
When Curlews cry beneath the Village-walls,
And to her straggling Brood the Partridge calls;
Their shortliv'd Jubilee the Creatures keep,
Which but endures, whilst Tyrant-Man does sleep:
When a sedate Content the Spirit feels,
And no fierce Light disturbs, whilst it reveals;
But silent Musings urge the Mind to seek
Something, too high for Syllables to speak;
Till the free Soul to a compos'dness charm'd,
Finding the Elements of Rage disarm'd,
O'er all below a solemn Quiet grown,
Joys in th' inferiour World, and thinks it like her Own:
In such a Night let Me abroad remain,
Till Morning breaks, and All's confus'd again;
Our Cares, our Toils, our Clamours are renew'd,
Or Pleasures, seldom reach'd, again pursu'd.

Petrarch
ODE 17

From thought to thought, from mountain peak to mountain
Love leads me on; for I can never still
My trouble on the world's well-beaten ways.
If on a barren heath there springs a fountain,
Or a dark valley huddles under a hill,
There may the grieving soul find quiet days;
There freely she obeys
Love's orders, laughing, weeping, hoping, fearing,
And the face writes a gloss upon the soul
Now glad, now charged with dole,
Not long in my manner persevering.
At sight of me a man of subtle wit
Would say, "He burns, and sees no end of it."

In the high mountains, in the woods I find
A little solace; every haunt of man
Is to my mood a mortal enemy.
At every step a new thought comes to mind
Of my dear lady, whose remembrance can
Turn all the hurt of love to gayety.
I would no sooner be
Quit of this bittersweet existence here,
Than I reflect, "Yet even now Love may
Destine the better day;
I, loathing self, may be to others dear!"
So I go thinking, hoping, sighing, now;
May it be true indeed? And when? And how?

And in the shade of a pine tree on a hill

I halt, and all the tumbled rocks near by
Are pictured with the beauty of her face;
And tears of tender melancholy fill
My bosom; and "Alas! alas!" I cry,
"What have I come to! From how far a place!"
But, for the little space
That the uneasy mind thus looks on her,
Rapt out of self into another sphere,
Then I feel Love so near
That the tricked soul rejoices it should err.
So dear I see her, and so fair and pure
That I pray only that the fraud endure.

Often I've seen her—who'll believe me now?
Treading the grass, cleaving the lucid water,
Alive, alive, in a forest beech-trunk caught,
White mid the clouds; so fair, Leda would vow
The famous beauty of her lovely daughter
Is dimmed as a star when the broad sun beams hot.
And, in what savage spot
I chance to be, in what most barren shore,
Ever more beautiful she walks with me.
Then, when Truth makes to flee
My darling cheat, I find my self once more
A dead stone statue, set on living stone,
Of one who thinks and grieves and writes alone.

Now it's my whole desire and all my pleasure
Up to the highest mountain-pass to climb
To dizzy and unshadowed solitude,
And thence I send my flying gaze to measure
My length of woe; I weep a little time;
The mist of grief blows from my dismal mood.
I stare afar and brood

On the leagues that lie between me and that face,
Ever so near and yet so far away.
Soft to myself I say,
"My soul, be brave; perhaps, in that far place,
She thinks of you in absence, and she sighs!"
And my soul suddenly wakes and gladly cries.

My song, beyond these alps,
In the land where skies are gladder and more clear,
You'll see me soon, where a quick streamlet flows,
And where the fragrance blows
Of the fresh laurel that I love so dear.
There is my heart, and she who reft it me;
Here you may see only my effigy.

William Hazlitt
ON GOING A JOURNEY

One of the pleasantest things in the world is going a journey; but I like to go by myself. I can enjoy society in a room; but out of doors, nature is company enough for me. I am then never less alone than when alone.

"The fields his study, nature was his book."

I cannot see the wit of walking and talking at the same time. When I am in the country, I wish to vegetate like the country. I am not for criticising hedge-rows and black cattle. I go out of town in order to forget the town and all that is in it. There are those who for this purpose go to watering-places, and carry the metropolis with them. I like more elbow-room, and fewer incumbrances. I like solitude, when I give myself up to it, for the sake of solitude; nor do I ask for

—"a friend in my retreat,
Whom I may whisper solitude is sweet."

The soul of a journey is liberty, perfect liberty, to think, feel, do just as one pleases. We go a journey chiefly to be free of all impediments and of all inconveniences; to leave ourselves behind, much more to get rid of others. It is because I want a little breathing-space to muse on indifferent matters, where Contemplation

"May plume her feathers and let grow her wings,
That in the various bustle of resort
Were all too ruffled, and sometimes impair'd,"

that I absent myself from the town for awhile, without feeling at a loss the moment I am left by myself. Instead of a friend in a postchaise or in a tilbury, to exchange good things with, and vary the same stale topics over again, for once let me have a truce with impertinence. Give me the clear blue sky over my head, and the green turf beneath my feet, a winding road before me, and a three hours' march to dinner—and then to thinking! It is hard if I cannot start some game on these lone heaths. I laugh, I run, I leap, I sing for joy. From the point of yonder rolling cloud, I plunge into my past being, and revel there, as the sunburnt Indian plunges headlong into the wave that wafts him to his native shore. Then long-forgotten things, like "sunken wrack and sumless treasuries," burst upon my eager sight, and I begin to feel, think, and be myself again. Instead of an awkward silence, broken by attempts at wit or dull com-mon-places, mine is that undisturbed silence of the heart which alone is per-fect eloquence. No one likes puns, alliterations, antitheses, argument, and analysis better than I do; but I sometimes had rather be without them. "Leave, oh, leave me to my repose!" I have just now other business in hand, which would seem idle to you, but is with me "the very stuff of the conscience." Is not this wild rose sweet without a comment? Does not this daisy leap to my heart, set in its coat of emerald? Yet if I were to explain to you the circumstance that has so endeared it to me, you would only smile. Had I not better then keep it to myself, and let it serve me to brood over, from here to yonder craggy point, and from thence onward to the far-distant horizon? I should be but bad company all that way, and therefore prefer being alone. I have heard it said that you may, when the moody fit comes on, walk or ride on by yourself, and indulge your reveries. But this looks like a breach of manners, a neglect of oth-ers, and you are thinking all the time that you ought to rejoin your party. "Out upon such half-faced fellowship," say I. I like to be either entirely to myself, or entirely at the disposal of others; to talk or be silent, to walk or sit still, to be sociable or solitary. I was pleased with an observation of Mr Cobbet's, that "he thought it a bad French custom to drink our wine with our meals, and that an Englishman ought to do only one thing at a time." So I cannot talk and think, or indulge in melancholy musing and lively conversation by fits and starts. "Let me have a companion of my way," says Sterne, "were it but to remark how the shadows lengthen as the sun goes down." It is beautifully said: but in my opinion, this continual comparing of notes interferes with the involuntary impression of things upon the mind, and hurts the sentiment. If you only hint what you feel in a kind of dumb show, it is insipid; if you have to explain it, it is making a toil of a pleasure. You cannot read the book of nature, without being perpetually put to the trouble of translating it for the benefit of others. I am for the synthetical method on a journey, in preference to the analytical. I am content to lay in a stock of ideas then, and to examine and anatomise them afterwards. I want to see my vague notions float like the down of the thistle before the breeze, and not to have them entangled in the briars and thorns of controversy. For once, I like to have it all my own way; and this is impossible unless you are alone, or in such company as I do not covet. I have no objection to argue a point with any one for twenty miles of measured road, but not for pleasure. If you remark the scent of a beanfield crossing the road, perhaps your fellow-traveller has no smell. If you point to a distant object, perhaps he is short-sighted, and has to take out his glass to look at it. There is a feeling in the air, a tone in the colour of a cloud which hits your fancy, but the effect of which you are unprepared to account for. There is then no sympathy, but an uneasy craving after it, and a dissatisfaction which pursues you on the way, and in the end probably produces ill humour. Now I never quarrel with myself, and take all my own conclusions for granted till I find it necessary to defend them against objections. It is not merely that you may not be of accord on the objects and circumstances that present themselves before you—they may recall a number of ideas, and lead to associations too delicate and refined to be possibly communicated to others. Yet these I love to cherish, and some-times still fondly clutch them, when I can escape from the throng to do so. To give way to our feelings before company, seems extravagance or affectation; on the other hand, to have to unravel this mystery of our being at every turn, and to make others take an equal interest in it (otherwise the end is not answered) is a task to which few are competent. We must "give it an understanding, but no tongue." My old friend C—, however, could do both. He could go on in the most delightful explanatory way over hill and dale, a summer's day, and convert a landscape into a didactic poem or a Pindaric ode. "He talked far above singing." If I could so clothe my ideas in sounding and flowing words, I might perhaps wish to have some one with me to admire the swelling theme; or I could be more content, were it possible for me still to hear his echoing voice in the woods of All-Foxden. They had "that fine madness in them which our first poets had;" and if they could have been caught by some rare instrument, would have breathed such strains as the following.

> —"Here be woods as green
> As any, air likewise as fresh and sweet
> As when smooth Zephyrus plays on the fleet
> Face of the curled stream, with flow'rs as many
> As the young spring gives, and as choice as any;
> Here be all new delights, cool streams and wells,
> Arbours o'ergrown with woodbine, caves and dells:
> Choose where thou wilt, while I sit by and sing,
> Or gather rushes to make many a ring
> For thy long fingers; tell thee tales of love,
> How the pale Phoebe, hunting in a grove,
> First saw the boy Endymion, from whose eyes
> She took eternal fire that never dies;
> How she convey'd him softly in a sleep,
> His temples bound with poppy, to the steep
> Head of old Latmos, where she stoops each night,
> Gilding the mountain with her brother's light,
> To kiss her sweetest"—
>   FAITHFUL SHEPHERDESS.

Had I words and images at command like these, I would attempt to wake the thoughts that lie slumbering on golden ridges in the evening clouds: but at the sight of nature my fancy, poor as it is, droops and closes up its leaves, like flowers at sunset. I can make nothing out on the spot: —I must have time to collect myself.

In general, a good thing spoils out-of-door prospects: it should be reserved for Table-talk. L— is for this reason, I take it, the worst company in the world out of doors; because he is the best within. I grant, there is one subject on which it is pleasant to talk on a journey; and that is, what one shall have for supper when we get to our inn at night. The open air improves this sort of conversation or friendly altercation, by setting a keener edge on appetite. Every mile of the road heightens the flavour of the viands we expect at the end of it. How fine it is to enter some old town, walled and turreted, just at the approach of night-fall, or to come to some straggling village, with the lights streaming through the surrounding gloom; and then after inquiring for the best entertainment that the place affords, to "take one's ease at one's inn!" These eventful moments in our lives are in fact too precious, too full of solid, heart-felt happiness to be frittered and dribbled away in imperfect sympathy. I would have them all to myself, and drain them to the last drop: they will do to talk of or to write about afterwards. What a delicate speculation it is, after drinking whole goblets of tea,

"The cups that cheer, but not inebriate,"

and letting the fumes ascend into the brain, to sit considering what we shall have for supper—eggs and a rasher, a rabbit smothered in onions, or an excellent veal-cutlet! Sancho in such a situation once fixed upon cow-heel; and his choice, though he could not help it, is not to be disparaged. Then in the intervals of pictured scenery and Shandean contemplation, to catch the preparation and the stir in the kitchen—*Procul, O procul este profani!* These hours are sacred to silence and to musing, to be treasured up in the memory, and to feed the source of smiling thoughts hereafter. I would not waste them in idle talk; or if I must have the integrity of fancy broken in upon, I would rather it were by a stranger than a friend. A stranger takes his hue and character from the time and place; he is a part of the furniture and costume of an inn. If he is a Quaker, or from the West Riding of Yorkshire, so much the better. I do not even try to sympathise with him, and *he breaks no squares.* I associate nothing with my travelling companion but present objects and passing events. In his ignorance of me and my affairs, I in a manner forget myself. But a friend reminds one of other things, rips up old grievances, and destroys the abstraction of the scene. He comes in ungraciously between us and our imaginary character. Something is dropped in the course of conversation that gives a hint of your profession and pursuits; or from having some one with you that knows the less sublime portions of your history, it seems that other people do. You are no longer a citizen of the world: but your "unhoused free condition is put into circumscription and confine." The *incognito* of an inn is one of its striking privileges—"lord of one's-self, uncumber'd with a name." Oh! it is great to shake off the trammels of the world and of public opinion—to lose our importunate, tormenting, everlasting personal identity in the elements of nature, and become the creature of the moment, clear of all ties—to hold to the universe only by a dish of sweet-breads, and to owe nothing but the score of the evening—and no longer seeking for applause and meeting with contempt, to be known by no other title than *the Gentleman in the parlour!* One may take one's choice of all characters in this romantic state of uncertainty as to one's real pretensions, and become indefinitely respectable and negatively right-worshipful. We baffle prejudice and disappoint conjecture; and from being so to others, begin to be objects of curiosity and wonder even to ourselves. We are no more those hackneyed commonplaces that we appear in the world: an inn restores us to the level of nature, and quits scores with society! I have certainly spent some enviable hours at inns—sometimes when I have been left entirely to myself, and have tried to solve some metaphysical problem, as once at Witham-common, where I found out the proof that likeness is not a case of the association of ideas—at other times, when there have been pictures in the room, as at St Neot's, (I think it was) where I first met with Gribelin's engravings of the Cartoons, into which I entered at once; and at a little inn on the borders of Wales, where there happened to be hanging some of Westall's drawings, which I compared triumphantly (for a theory that I had, not for the admired artist) with the figure of a girl who had ferried me over the Severn, standing up in the boat between me and the fading twilight—at other times I might mention luxuriating in books, with a peculiar interest in this way, as I remember sitting up half the night to read *Paul and Virginia,* which I picked up at an inn at Bridgewater, after being drenched in the rain all day; and at the same place I got through two volumes of Madame D'Arblay's *Camilla.* It was on the tenth of April, 1798, that I sat down to a volume of the *New Eloise,* at the inn at Llangollen, over a bottle of sherry and a cold chicken. The letter I chose was that in which St Preux describes his feelings as he first caught a glimpse from the heights of the Jura of the Pays de Vaud, which I had brought with me as a *bonne bouche* to crown the evening with. It was my birthday, and I had for the first time come from a place in the neighbourhood to visit this delightful spot. The road to Llangollen turns off between Chirk and Wrexham; and on passing a certain point, you come all at once upon the valley, which opens like an amphitheatre, broad, barren hills rising in majestic state on either side, with "green upland swells that echo to the bleat of flocks" below, and the river Dee babbling over its stony bed in the midst of them. The valley at this time "glittered green with sunny showers," and a budding ash-tree dipped its tender branches in the chiding stream. How proud, how glad I was to walk along the high road that commanded the delicious prospect, repeating the lines which I have just quoted from Mr Coleridge's poems! But besides the prospect which opened beneath my feet, another also opened to my inward sight, a heavenly vision, on which were written, in letters large as Hope could make them, these four words, LIBERTY, GENIUS, LOVE, VIRTUE; which have since faded into the light of common day, or mock my idle gaze.

"The beautiful is vanished, and returns not."

Still I would return some time or other to this enchanted spot; but I would return to it alone. What other self could I find to share that influx of thoughts, of regret, and delight, the traces of which I could hardly conjure up to myself, so much have they been broken and defaced! I could stand on some tall rock, and overlook the precipice of years that separates me from what I then was. I was at that time going shortly to visit the poet whom I have above named. Where is he now? Not only I myself have changed; the world, which was then new to me, has become old and incorrigible. Yet will I turn to thee in thought, O sylvan Dee, as then thou wert, in joy, in youth and gladness; and thou shalt always be to me the river of Paradise, where I will drink of the waters of life freely!

There is hardly any thing that shows the short-sightedness or capricious-ness of the imagination more than travelling does. With change of place we change our ideas; nay, our opinions and feelings. We can by an effort indeed transport ourselves to old and long-forgotten scenes, and then the picture of the mind revives again; but we forget those that we have just left. It seems that we can think but of one place at a time. The canvas of the fancy has only a cer-tain extent, and if we paint one set of objects upon it, they immediately efface every other. We cannot enlarge our conceptions; we only shift our point of view. The landscape bares its bosom to the enraptured eye; we take our fill of it; and seem as if we could form no other image of beauty or grandeur. We pass on, and think no more of it: the horizon that shuts it from our sight also blots it from our memory like a dream. In travelling through a wild barren country, I can form no idea of a woody and cultivated one. It appears to me that all the world must be barren, like what I see of it. In the country we forget the town, and in town we despise the country. "Beyond Hyde Park," says Sir Fopling Flutter, "all is a desert." All that part of the map that we do not see before us is a blank. The world in our conceit of it is not much bigger than a nutshell. It is not one prospect expanded into another, county joined to county, kingdom to kingdom, lands to seas, making an image voluminous and vast; —the mind can form no larger idea of space than the eye can take in at a single glance. The rest is a name written on a map, a calculation of arithmetic. For instance, what is the true signification of that immense mass of territory and population, known by the name of China to us? An inch of paste-board on a wooden globe, of no more account than a China orange! Things near us are seen the size of life: things at a distance are diminished to the size of understanding. We measure the universe by ourselves, and even comprehend the texture of our own being only piece-meal. In this way, however, we remember an infinity of things and places. The mind is like a mechanical instrument that plays a great variety of tunes, but it must play them in succession. One idea recalls another, but it at the same time excludes all others. In trying to renew old recollections, we cannot as it were unfold the whole web of our existence; we must pick out the single threads. So in coming to a place where we have formerly lived and with which we have intimate associations, every one must have found that the feeling grows more vivid the nearer we approach the spot, from the mere anticipation of the actual impression: we remember circumstances, feelings, persons, faces, names, that we had not thought of for years; but for the time all the rest of the world is forgotten! —To return to the question I have quitted above.

I have no objection to go to see ruins, aqueducts, pictures, in company with a friend or a party, but rather the contrary, for the former reason reversed. They are intelligible matters, and will bear talking about. The sentiment here is not tacit, but communicable and overt. Salisbury Plain is barren of criticism, but Stonehenge will bear a discussion antiquarian, picturesque, and philosophical. In setting out on a party of pleasure, the first consideration always is where we shall go: in taking a solitary ramble, the question is what we shall meet with by the way. The mind then is "its own place;" nor are we anxious to arrive at the end of our journey. I can myself do the honours indifferently well to works of art and curiosity. I once took a party to Oxford with no mean *éclat*—shewed them the seat of the Muses at a distance,

"With glistering spires and pinnacles adorn'd"—

descanted on the learned air that breathes from the grassy quadrangles and stone walls of halls and colleges—was at home in the Bodleian; and at Blenheim quite superseded the powdered Cicerone that attended us, and that pointed in vain with his wand to common-place beauties in matchless pictures. —As another exception to the above reasoning, I should not feel confident in venturing on a journey in a foreign country without a companion. I should want at intervals to hear the sound of my own language. There is an involuntary antipathy in the mind of an Englishman to foreign manners and notions that requires the assistance of social sympathy to carry it off. As the distance from home increases, this relief, which was at first a luxury, becomes a passion and an appetite. A person would almost feel stifled to find himself in the deserts of Arabia without friends and countrymen: there must be allowed to be something in the view of Athens or old Rome that claims the utterance of speech; and I own that the Pyramids are too mighty for any single contemplation. In such situations, so opposite to all one's ordinary train of ideas, one seems a species by one's-self, a limb torn off from society, unless one can meet with instant fellowship and support. —Yet I did not feel this want or craving very pressing once, when I first set my foot on the laughing shores of France. Calais was peopled with novelty and delight. The confused, busy murmur of the place was like oil and wine poured into my ears; nor did the mariners' hymn, which was sung from the top of an old crazy vessel in the harbour, as the sun went down, send an alien sound into my soul. I breathed the air of general humanity. I walked over "the vine-covered hills and gay regions of France," erect and satisfied; for the image of man was not cast down and chained to the foot of arbitrary thrones. I was at no loss for language, for that of all the great schools of painting was open to me. The whole is vanished like a shade. Pictures, heroes, glory, freedom, all are fled: nothing remains but the Bourbons and the French people! —There is undoubtedly a sensation in travelling into foreign parts that is to be had nowhere else: but it is more pleasing at the time than lasting. It is too remote from our habitual associations to be a common topic of discourse or reference, and, like a dream or another state of existence, does not piece into our daily modes of life. It is an animated but a momentary hallucination. It demands an effort to exchange our actual for our ideal identity; and to feel the pulse of our old transports revive very keenly, we must "jump" all our present comforts and connexions. Our romantic and itinerant character is not to be domesticated. Dr Johnson remarked how little foreign travel added to the facilities of conversation in those who had been abroad. In fact, the time we have spent there is both delightful and in one sense instructive; but it appears to be cut out of our substantial, downright existence, and never to join kindly on to it. We are not the same, but another, and perhaps more enviable individual, all the time we are out of our own country. We are lost to ourselves, as well as to our friends. So the poet somewhat quaintly sings,

"Out of my country and myself I go."

Those who wish to forget painful thoughts, do well to absent themselves for a while from the ties and objects that recall them: but we can be said only to fulfil our destiny in the place that gave us birth. I should on this account like well enough to spend the whole of my life in travelling abroad, if I could any where borrow another life to spend afterwards at home!

Ursula K. Le Guin
THE ONES WHO WALK AWAY FROM OMELAS

With a clamor of bells that set the swallows soaring, the Festival of Summer came to the city Omelas, bright-towered by the sea. The rigging of the boats in harbor sparkled with flags. In the streets between houses with red roofs and painted walls, between old moss-grown gardens and under avenues of trees, past great parks and public buildings, processions moved. Some were decorous: old people in long stiff robes of mauve and grey, grave master workmen, quiet, merry women carrying their babies and chatting as they walked. In other streets the music beat faster, a shimmering of gong and tambourine, and the people went dancing, the procession was a dance. Children dodged in and out, their high calls rising like the swallows' crossing flights over the music and the singing. All the processions wound towards the north side of the city, where on the great water-meadow called the Green Fields boys and girls, naked in the bright air, with mudstained feet and ankles and long, lithe arms, exercised their restive horses before the race. The horses wore no gear at all but a halter without bit. Their manes were braided with streamers of silver, gold, and green. They flared their nostrils and pranced and boasted to one another; they were vastly excited, the horse being the only animal who has adopted our ceremonies as his own. Far off to the north and west the mountains stood up half encircling Omelas on her bay. The air of morning was so clear that the snow still crowning the Eighteen Peaks burned with white-gold fire across the miles of sunlit air, under the dark blue of the sky. There was just enough wind to make the banners that marked the racecourse snap and flutter now and then. In the silence of the broad green meadows one could hear the music winding through the city streets, farther and nearer and ever approaching, a cheerful faint sweetness of the air that from time to time trembled and gathered together and broke out into the great joyous clanging of the bells.

Joyous! How is one to tell about joy? How describe the citizens of Omelas?

They were not simple folk, you see, though they were happy. But we do not say the words of cheer much any more. All smiles have become archaic. Given a description such as this one tends to make certain assumptions. Given a description such as this one tends to look next for the King, mounted on a splendid stallion and surrounded by his noble knights, or perhaps in a golden litter borne by great-muscled slaves. But there was no king. They did not use swords, or keep slaves. They were not barbarians. I do not know the rules and laws of their society, but I suspect that they were singularly few. As they did without monarchy and slavery, so they also go on without the stock exchange, the advertisement, the secret police, and the bomb. Yet I repeat that these were not simple folk, not dulcet shepherds, noble savages, bland utopians. They were not less complex than us. The trouble is that we have a bad habit, encouraged by pedants and sophisticates, of considering happiness as something rather stupid. Only pain is intellectual, only evil interesting. This is the treason of the artist: a refusal to admit the banality of evil and the terrible boredom of pain. If you can't lick 'em, join 'em. If it hurts, repeat it. But to praise despair is to condemn delight, to embrace violence is to lose hold of everything else. We have almost lost hold; we can no longer describe a happy man, nor make any celebration of joy. How can I tell you about the people of Omelas? They were not naive and happy children—though their children were, in fact, happy. They were mature, intelligent, passionate adults whose lives were not wretched. O miracle! but I wish I could describe it better. I wish I could convince you. Omelas sounds in my words like a city in a fairy tale, long ago and far away, once upon a time. Perhaps it would be best if you imagined it as your own fancy bids, assuming it will rise to the occasion, for certainly I cannot suit you all. For instance, how about technology? I think that there would be no cars or helicopters in and above the streets; this follows from the fact that the people of Omelas are happy people. Happiness is based on a just discrimination of what is necessary, what is neither necessary nor destructive, and what is destructive. In the middle category, however—that of the unnecessary but undestructive, that of comfort, luxury, exuberance, etc.—they could perfectly well have central heating, subway trains, washing machines, and all kinds of marvelous devices not yet invented here, floating light-sources, fuelless power, a cure for the common cold. Or they could have none of that: it doesn't matter. As you like it. I incline to think that people from towns up and down the coast have been coming in to Omelas during the last days before the Festival on very fast little trains and double-decked trams, and that the train station of Omelas is actually the handsomest building in town, though plainer than the magnificent Farmers' Market. But even granted trains, I fear that Omelas so far strikes some of you as goody-goody. Smiles, bells, parades, horses, bleh. If so, please add an orgy. If an orgy would help, don't hesitate. Let us not, however, have temples from which issue beautiful nude priests and priestesses already half in ecstasy and ready to copulate with any man or woman, lover or stranger, who desires union with the deep godhead of the blood, although that was my first idea. But really it would be better not to have any temples in Omelas—at least, not manned temples. Religion yes, clergy no. Surely the beautiful nudes can just wander about, offering themselves like divine soufflés to the hunger of the needy and the rapture of the flesh. Let them join the processions. Let tambourines be struck above the copulations, and the glory of desire be proclaimed upon the gongs, and (a not unimportant point) let the offspring of these delightful rituals be beloved and looked after by all. One thing I know there is none of in Omelas is guilt. But what else should there be? I thought at first there were no drugs, but that is puritanical. For those who like it, the faint insistent sweetness of *drooz* may perfume the ways of the city, *drooz* which first brings a great lightness and brilliance to the mind and limbs, and then after some hours a dreamy languor, and wonderful visions at last of the very arcana and inmost secrets of the Universe, as well as exciting the pleasure of sex beyond all belief; and it is not habit-forming. For more modest tastes I think there ought to be beer. What else, what else belongs in the joyous city? The sense of victory, surely, the celebration of courage. But as we did without clergy, let us do without soldiers. The joy built upon successful slaughter is not the right kind of joy; it will not do; it is fearful and it is trivial. A boundless and generous contentment, a magnanimous triumph felt not against some outer enemy but in communion with the finest and fairest in the souls of all men everywhere and the splendor of the world's summer: this is what swells the hearts of the people of Omelas, and the victory they celebrate is that of life. I really don't think many of them need to take *drooz*.

Most of the processions have reached the Green Fields by now. A marvelous smell of cooking goes forth from the red and blue tents of the provisioners. The faces of small children are amiably sticky; in the benign grey beard of a man a couple of crumbs of rich pastry are entangled. The youths and girls have mounted their horses and are beginning to group around the starting line of the course. An old woman, small, fat, and laughing, is passing out flowers from a basket, and tall young men wear her flowers in their shining hair. A child of nine or ten sits at the edge of the crowd, alone, playing on a wooden flute. People pause to listen, and they smile, but they do not speak to him, for he never ceases playing and never sees them, his dark eyes wholly rapt in the sweet, thin magic of the tune.

He finishes, and slowly lowers his hands holding the wooden flute.

As if that little private silence were the signal, all at once a trumpet sounds from the pavilion near the starting line: imperious, melancholy, piercing. The horses rear on their slender legs, and some of them neigh in answer. Sober-faced, the young riders stroke the horses' necks and soothe them, whispering, "Quiet, quiet, there my beauty, my hope. . . ." They begin to form in rank along the starting line. The crowds along the racecourse are like a field of grass and flowers in the wind. The Festival of Summer has begun.

Do you believe? Do you accept the festival, the city, the joy? No? Then let me describe one more thing.

In a basement under one of the beautiful public buildings of Omelas, or perhaps in the cellar of one of its spacious private homes, there is a room. It has one locked door, and no window. A little light seeps in dustily between cracks in the boards, secondhand from a cobwebbed window somewhere across the cellar. In one corner of the little room a couple of mops, with stiff, clotted, foul-smelling heads, stand near a rusty bucket. The floor is dirt, a little damp to the touch, as cellar dirt usually is. The room is about three paces long and two wide: a mere broom closet or disused tool room. In the room a child is sitting. It could be a boy or a girl. It looks about six, but actually is nearly ten. It is feeble-minded. Perhaps it was born defective, or perhaps it has become imbecile through fear, malnutrition, and neglect. It picks its nose and occasionally fumbles vaguely with its toes or genitals, as it sits hunched in the corner farthest from the bucket and the two mops. It is afraid of the mops. It finds them horrible. It shuts its eyes, but it knows the mops are still standing there; and the door is locked; and nobody will come. The door is always locked; and nobody ever comes, except that sometimes—the child has no understanding of time or interval—sometimes the door rattles terribly and opens, and a person, or several people, are there. One of them may come in and kick the child to make it stand up. The others never come close, but peer in at it with frightened, disgusted eyes. The food bowl and the water jug are hastily filled, the door is locked, the eyes disappear. The people at the door never say anything, but the child, who has not always lived in the tool room, and can remember sunlight and its mother's voice, sometimes speaks. "I will be good," it says. "Please let me out. I will be good!" They never answer. The child used to scream for help at night, and cry a good deal, but now it only makes a kind of whining, "eh-haa, eh-haa," and it speaks less and less often. It is so thin there are no calves to its legs; its belly protrudes; it lives on a half-bowl of corn meal and grease a day. It is naked. Its buttocks and thighs are a mass of festered sores, as it sits in its own excrement continually.

They all know it is there, all the people of Omelas. Some of them have come to see it, others are content merely to know it is there. They all know that it has to be there. Some of them understand why, and some do not, but they all understand that their happiness, the beauty of their city, the tenderness of their friendships, the health of their children, the wisdom of their scholars, the skill of their makers, even the abundance of their harvests and the kindly weathers of their skies, depend wholly on this child's abominable misery.

This is usually explained to children when they are between eight and twelve, whenever they seem capable of understanding; and most of those who come to see the child are young people, though often enough an adult comes, or comes back, to see the child. No matter how well the matter has been explained to them, these young spectators are always shocked and sickened at the sight. They feel disgust, which they had thought themselves superior to. They feel anger, outrage, impotence, despite all the explanations. They would like to do something for the child. But there is nothing they can do. If the child were brought up into the sunlight out of that vile place, if it were cleaned and fed and comforted, that would be a good thing, indeed; but if it were done, in that day and hour all the prosperity and beauty and delight of Omelas would wither and be destroyed. Those are the terms. To exchange all the goodness and grace of every life in Omelas for that single, small improvement: to throw away the happiness of thousands for the chance of the happiness of one: that would be to let guilt within the walls indeed.

The terms are strict and absolute; there may not even be a kind word spoken to the child.

Often the young people go home in tears, or in a tearless rage, when they have seen the child and faced this terrible paradox. They may brood over it for weeks or years. But as time goes on they begin to realize that even if the child could be released, it would not get much good of its freedom: a little vague pleasure of warmth and food, no doubt, but little more. It is too degraded and imbecile to know any real joy. It has been afraid too long ever to be free of fear. Its habits are too uncouth for it to respond to humane treatment. Indeed, after so long it would probably be wretched without walls about it to protect it, and darkness for its eyes, and its own excrement to sit in. Their tears at the bitter injustice dry when they begin to perceive the terrible justice of reality, and to accept it. Yet it is their tears and anger, the trying of their generosity and the acceptance of their helplessness, which are perhaps the true source of the splendor of their lives. Theirs is no vapid, irresponsible happiness. They know that they, like the child, are not free. They know compassion. It is the existence of the child, and their knowledge of its existence, that makes possible the nobility of their architecture, the poignancy of their music, the profundity of their science. It is because of the child that they are so gentle with children. They know that if the wretched one were not there snivelling in the dark, the other one, the flute-player, could make no joyful music as the young riders line up in their beauty for the race in the sunlight of the first morning of summer.

Now do you believe in them? Are they not more credible? But there is one more thing to tell, and this is quite incredible.

At times one of the adolescent girls or boys who go to see the child does not go home to weep or rage, does not, in fact, go home at all. Sometimes also a man or woman much older falls silent for a day or two, and then leaves home. These people go out into the street, and walk down the street alone. They keep walking, and walk straight out of the city of Omelas, through the beautiful gates. They keep walking across the farmlands of Omelas. Each one goes alone, youth or girl, man or woman. Night falls; the traveler must pass down village streets, between the houses with yellow-lit windows, and on into the darkness of the fields. Each alone, they go west or north, towards the mountains. They go on. They leave Omelas, they walk ahead into the darkness, and they do not come back. The place they go towards is a place even less imaginable to most of us than the city of happiness. I cannot describe it at all. It is possible that it does not exist. But they seem to know where they are going, the ones who walk away from Omelas.

Rainer Maria Rilke
ORPHEUS, EURYDICE AND HERMES

Translated by Robert Lowell

That's the strange regalia of souls.
Vibrant
as platinum filaments they went,
like arteries through their darkness. From the holes
of powder beetles, from the otter's bed,
from the oak king judging by the royal oak—
blood like our own life-blood, sprang.
Otherwise nothing was red.

The dark was heavier than Caesar's foot.

There were canyons there,
distracted forests, and bridges over air-pockets;
a great gray, blind lake
mooned over the background canals,
like a bag of winds over the Caucasus.
Through terraced highlands, stocked with cattle and patience,
streaked the single road.
It was unwinding like a bandage.

They went on this road.

First the willowy man in the blue cloak;
he didn't say a thing. He counted his toes.
His step ate up the road,
a yard at a time, without bruising a thistle. His hands fell,

clammy and clenched,
as if they feared the folds of his tunic,
as if they didn't know a thing about the frail lyre,
hooked on his left shoulder,
like roses wrestling an olive tree.

It was as though his intelligence were cut in two.
His outlook worried like a dog behind him,
now diving ahead, now romping back,
now yawning on its haunches at an elbow of the road.
What he heard breathed myrrh behind him,
and often it seemed to reach back to them,
those two others
on oath to follow behind to the finish.
Then again there was nothing behind him,
only the backring of his heel,
and the currents of air in his blue cloak.
He said to himself, "For all that, they are there."
He spoke aloud and heard his own voice die.
"They are coming, but if they are two,
how fearfully light their step is!"
Couldn't he turn round? (Yet a single back-look
would be the ruin of this work
so near perfection.) And as a matter of fact,
he knew he must now turn to them, those two light ones,
who followed and kept their counsel.
First the road-god, the messenger man . . .
His caduceus shadow-bowing behind him,
his eye arched, archaic,
his ankles feathered like arrows—
in his left hand he held *her,*
the one so loved that out of a single lyre
more sorrow came than from all women in labor,
so that out of this sorrow came
the fountain-head of the world: valleys, fields,

towns, roads . . . acropolis,
marble quarries, goats, vineyards.
And this sorrow-world circled about her,
just as the sun and stern stars
circle the earth—
a heaven of anxiety ringed by the determined stars . . .
that's how *she* was.

She leant, however, on the god's arm;
her step was delicate from her wound—
uncertain, drugged and patient.
She was drowned in herself, as in a higher hope,
and she didn't give the man in front of her a thought,
nor the road climbing to life.
She was in herself. Being dead
fulfilled her beyond fulfillment.
Like an apple full of sugar and darkness,
she was full of her decisive death,
so green she couldn't bite into it.
She was still in her marble maidenhood,
untouchable. Her sex had closed house,
like a young flower rebuking the night air.
Her hands were still ringing and tingling—
even the light touch of the god
was almost a violation.

A woman?
She was no longer that blond transcendence
so often ornamenting the singer's meters,
nor a hanging garden in his double bed.
She had wearied of being the hero's one possession.

She was as bountiful as uncoiled hair,
poured out like rain,
shared in a hundred pieces like her wedding cake.

She was a root, self-rooted.

And when the god suddenly gripped her,
and said with pain in his voice, "He is looking back at us,"
she didn't get through to the words,
and answered vaguely, "Who?"

Far there, dark against the clear entrance,
stood some one, or rather no one
you'd ever know. He stood and stared
at the one level, inevitable road,
as the reproachful god of messengers
looking round, pushed off again.
His caduceus was like a shotgun on his shoulder.

Ray Bradbury
THE PEDESTRIAN

To enter out into that silence that was the city at eight o'clock of a misty evening in November, to put your feet upon that buckling concrete walk, to step over grassy seams and make your way, hands in pockets, through the silences, that was what Mr. Leonard Mead most dearly loved to do. He would stand upon the corner of an intersection and peer down long moonlit avenues of sidewalk in four directions, deciding which way to go, but it really made no difference; he was alone in this world of 2053 A.D., or as good as alone, and with a final decision made, a path selected, he would stride off, sending patterns of frosty air before him like the smoke of a cigar.

Sometimes he would walk for hours and miles and return only at midnight to his house. And on his way he would see the cottages and homes with their dark windows, and it was not unequal to walking through a graveyard where only the faintest glimmers of firefly light appeared in flickers behind the windows. Sudden gray phantoms seemed to manifest upon inner room walls where a curtain was still undrawn against the night, or there were whisperings and murmurs where a window in a tomblike building was still open.

Mr. Leonard Mead would pause, cock his head, listen, look, and march on, his feet making no noise on the lumpy walk. For long ago he had wisely changed to sneakers when strolling at night, because the dogs in intermittent squads would parallel his journey with barkings if he wore hard heels, and lights might click on and faces appear and an entire street be startled by the passing of a lone figure, himself, in the early November evening.

On this particular evening he began his journey in a westerly direction, toward the hidden sea. There was a good crystal frost in the air; it cut the nose and made the lungs blaze like a Christmas tree inside; you could feel the cold light going on and off, all the branches filled with invisible snow. He listened to the faint push of his soft shoes through autumn leaves with satisfaction, and whistled a cold quiet whistle between his teeth, occasionally picking up a leaf as he passed, examining its skeletal pattern in the infrequent lamplights as he went on, smelling its rusty smell.

"Hello, in there," he whispered to every house on every side as he moved. "What's up tonight on Channel 4, Channel 7, Channel 9? Where are the cowboys rushing, and do I see the United States Cavalry over the next hill to the rescue?"

The street was silent and long and empty, with only his shadow moving like the shadow of a hawk in mid-country. If he closed his eyes and stood very still, frozen, he could imagine himself upon the center of a plain, a wintry, windless Arizona desert with no house in a thousand miles, and only dry river beds, the streets, for company.

"What is it now?" he asked the houses, noticing his wrist watch. "Eight-thirty P.M.? Time for a dozen assorted murders? A quiz? A revue? A comedian falling off the stage?"

Was that a murmur of laughter from within a moon-white house? He hesitated, but went on when nothing more happened. He stumbled over a particularly uneven section of sidewalk. The cement was vanishing under flowers and grass. In ten years of walking by night or day for thousands of miles, he had never met another person walking, not one in all that time.

He came to a cloverleaf intersection which stood silent where two main highways crossed the town. During the day it was a thunderous surge of cars, the gas stations open, a great insect rustling and a ceaseless jockeying for position as the scarab-beetles, a faint incense puttering from their exhausts, skimmed homeward to the far directions. But now these highways, too, were like streams in a dry season, all stone and bed and moon radiance.

He turned back on a side street, circling around toward his home. He was within a block of his destination when the lone car turned a corner quite suddenly and flashed a fierce white cone of light upon him. He stood entranced, not unlike a night moth, stunned by the illumination, and then drawn toward it.

A metallic voice called to him:

"Stand still. Stay where you are! Don't move!"

He halted.

"Put up your hands!"

"But—" he said.

"Your hands up! Or we'll shoot!"

The police, of course, but what a rare, incredible thing; in a city of three million, there was only *one* police car left, wasn't that correct? Ever since a year ago, 2052, the election year, the force had been cut down from three cars to one. Crime was ebbing; there was no need now for the police, save for this one lone car wandering and wandering the empty streets.

"Your name?" said the police car in a metallic whisper. He couldn't see the men in it for the bright light in his eyes.

"Leonard Mead," he said.

"Speak up!"

"Leonard Mead!"

"Business or profession?"

"I guess you'd call me a writer."

"No profession," said the police car, as if talking to itself. The light held him fixed, like a museum specimen, needle thrust through chest.

"You might say that," said Mr. Mead. He hadn't written in years. Magazines and books didn't sell any more. Everything went on in the tomb-like houses at night now, he thought, continuing his fancy. The tombs, ill-lit by television light, where the people sat like the dead, the gray or multicolored lights touching their faces, but never really touching *them.*

"No profession," said the phonograph voice, hissing. "What are you doing out?"

"Walking," said Leonard Mead.

"Walking!"

"Just walking," he said simply, but his face felt cold.

"Walking, just walking, walking?"

"Yes, sir."

"Walking where? For what?"

"Walking for air, Walking to *see.*"

"Your address!"

"Eleven South Saint James Street."

"And there is air *in* your house, you have an air *conditioner,* Mr. Mead?"

"Yes."

"And you have a viewing screen in your house to see with?"

"No."

"No?" There was a crackling quiet that in itself was an accusation.

"Are you married, Mr. Mead?"

"No."

"Not married," said the police voice behind the fiery beam. The moon was high and clear among the stars and the houses were gray and silent.

"Nobody wanted me," said Leonard Mead with a smile.

"Don't speak unless you're spoken to!"

Leonard Mead waited in the cold night.

"Just *walking*, Mr. Mead?"

"Yes."

"But you haven't explained for what purpose."

"I explained; for air, and to see, and just to walk."

"Have you done this often?"

"Every night for years."

The police car sat in the center of the street with its radio throat faintly humming.

"Well, Mr. Mead," it said.

"Is that all?" he asked politely.

"Yes," said the voice. "Here." There was a sigh, a pop. The back door of the police car sprang wide. "Get in."

"Wait a minute, I haven't done anything!"

"Get in."

"I protest!"

"Mr. Mead."

He walked like a man suddenly drunk. As he passed the front window of the car he looked in. As he had expected, there was no one in the front seat, no one in the car at all.

"Get in."

He put his hand to the door and peered into the back seat, which was a little cell, a little black jail with bars. It smelled of riveted steel. It smelled of harsh antiseptic; it smelled too clean and hard and metallic. There was nothing soft there.

"Now if you had a wife to give you an alibi," said the iron voice. "But—"

"Where are you taking me?"

The car hesitated, or rather gave a faint whirring click, as if information, somewhere, was dropping card by punch-slotted card under electric eyes. "To the Psychiatric Center for Research on Regressive Tendencies."

He got in. The door shut with a soft thud. The police car rolled through the night avenues, flashing its dim lights ahead.

They passed one house on one street a moment later, one house in an entire city of houses that were dark, but this one particular house had all of its electric lights brightly lit, every window a loud yellow illumination, square and warm in the cool darkness.

"That's *my* house," said Leonard Mead.

No one answered him.

The car moved down the empty river-bed streets and off away, leaving the empty streets with the empty sidewalks, and no sound and no motion all the rest of the chill November night.

Jane Austen
FROM PERSUASION

It was a very fine November day, and the Miss Musgroves came through the little grounds, and stopped for no other purpose than to say, that they were going to take a long walk, and, therefore, concluded Mary could not like to go with them; and when Mary immediately replied, with some jealousy, at not being supposed a good walker, "Oh, yes, I should like to join you very much, I am very fond of a long walk;" Anne felt persuaded, by the looks of the two girls, that it was precisely what they did not wish, and admired again the sort of necessity which the family habits seemed to produce, of every thing being to be communicated, and every thing being to be done together, however undesired and inconvenient. She tried to dissuade Mary from going, but in vain; and that being the case, thought it best to accept the Miss Musgroves' much more cordial invitation to herself to go likewise, as she might be useful in turning back with her sister, and lessening the interference in any plan of their own.

"I cannot imagine why they should suppose I should not like a long walk," said Mary, as she went up stairs. "Every body is always supposing that I am not a good walker. And yet they would not have been pleased, if we had refused to join them. When people come in this manner on purpose to ask us, how can one say no?"

Just as they were setting off, the gentlemen returned. They had taken out a young dog, who had spoilt their sport, and sent them back early. Their time and strength, and spirits, were, therefore, exactly ready for this walk, and they entered into it with pleasure. Could Anne have foreseen such a junction, she would have staid at home; but, from some feelings of interest and curiosity, she fancied now that it was too late to retract, and the whole six set forward together in the direction chosen by the Miss Musgroves, who evidently considered the walk as under their guidance.

Anne's object was, not to be in the way of any body; and where the narrow paths across the fields made many separations necessary, to keep with her brother and sister. Her *pleasure* in the walk must arise from the exercise and the day, from the view of the last smiles of the year upon the tawny leaves and withered hedges, and from repeating to herself some few of the thousand poetical descriptions extant of autumn, that season of peculiar and inexhaustible influence on the mind of taste and tenderness, that season which has drawn from every poet, worthy of being read, some attempt at description, or some lines of feeling. She occupied her mind as much as possible in such like musings and quotations; but it was not possible, that when within reach of Captain Wentworth's conversation with either of the Miss Musgroves, she should not try to hear it; yet she caught little very remarkable. It was mere lively chat,—such as any young persons, on an intimate footing, might fall into. He was more engaged with Louisa than with Henrietta. Louisa certainly put more forward for his notice than her sister. This distinction appeared to increase, and there was one speech of Louisa's which struck her. After one of the many praises of the day, which were continually bursting forth, Captain Wentworth added: —

"What glorious weather for the Admiral and my sister! They meant to take a long drive this morning; perhaps we may hail them from some of these hills. They talked of coming into this side of the country. I wonder whereabouts they will upset to-day. Oh! it does happen very often, I assure you; but my sister makes nothing of it—she would as lieve be tossed out as not."

"Ah! You make the most of it, I know," cried Louisa, "but if it were really so, I should do just the same in her place. If I loved a man, as she loves the Admiral, I would always be with him, nothing should ever separate us, and I would rather be overturned by him, than driven safely by anybody else."

It was spoken with enthusiasm.

"Had you?" cried he, catching the same tone; "I honour you!" And there was silence between them for a little while.

Anne could not immediately fall into a quotation again. The sweet scenes of autumn were for a while put by—unless some tender sonnet, fraught with the apt analogy of the declining year, with declining happiness, and the images of youth and hope, and spring, all gone together, blessed her memory. She roused herself to say, as they struck by order into another path, "Is not this one of the ways to Winthrop?" But nobody heard, or, at least, nobody answered her.

Winthrop, however, or its environs—for young men are, sometimes to be met with, strolling about near home—was their destination; and after another half mile of gradual ascent through large enclosures, where the ploughs at work, and the fresh-made path spoke the farmer, counteracting the sweets of poetical despondence, and meaning to have spring again, they gained the summit of the most considerable hill, which parted Uppercross and Winthrop, and soon commanded a full view of the latter, at the foot of the hill on the other side.

Winthrop, without beauty and without dignity, was stretched before them; an indifferent house, standing low, and hemmed in by the barns and buildings of a farm-yard.

Mary exclaimed, "Bless me! here is Winthrop—I declare I had no idea!— Well now, I think we had better turn back; I am excessively tired."

Henrietta, conscious and ashamed, and seeing no cousin Charles walking along any path, or leaning against any gate, was ready to do as Mary wished; but "No!" said Charles Musgrove, and "No, no!" cried Louisa more eagerly, and taking her sister aside, seemed to be arguing the matter warmly.

Charles, in the meanwhile, was very decidedly declaring his resolution of calling on his aunt, now that he was so near; and very evidently, though more fearfully, trying to induce his wife to go too. But this was one of the points on which the lady shewed her strength, and when he recommended the advantage of resting herself a quarter of an hour at Winthrop, as she felt so tired, she resolutely answered, "Oh! no, indeed!—walking up that hill again would do her more harm than any sitting down could do her good;" and, in short, her look and manner declared, that go she would not.

After a little succession of these sort of debates and consultations, it was settled between Charles and his two sisters, that he and Henrietta should just run down for a few minutes, to see their aunt and cousins, while the rest of the party waited for them at the top of the hill. Louisa seemed the principal arranger of the plan; and, as she went a little way with them, down the hill, still talking to Henrietta, Mary took the opportunity of looking scornfully around her, and saying to Captain Wentworth—

"It is very unpleasant, having such connexions! But, I assure you, I have never been in the house above twice in my life."

She received no other answer, than an artificial, assenting smile, followed by a contemptuous glance, as he turned away, which Anne perfectly knew the meaning of.

The brow of the hill, where they remained, was a cheerful spot; Louisa returned, and Mary, finding a comfortable seat for herself on the step of a stile, was very well satisfied so long as the others all stood about her; but when Louisa drew Captain Wentworth away, to try for a gleaning of nuts in an adjoining hedge-row, and they were gone by degrees quite out of sight and sound, Mary was happy no longer; she quarrelled with her own seat—was sure Louisa had got a much better somewhere,—and nothing could prevent her from going to look for a better also. She turned through the same gate,—but could not see them.—Anne found a nice seat for her, on a dry sunny bank, under the hedge-row, in which she had no doubt of their still being, in some spot or other. Mary sat down for a moment, but it would not do; she was sure Louisa had found a better seat somewhere else, and she would go on till she overtook her.

Anne, really tired herself, was glad to sit down; and she very soon heard Captain Wentworth and Louisa in the hedge-row, behind her, as if making their way back, along the rough, wild sort of channel, down the centre. They were speaking as they drew near. Louisa's voice was the first distinguished. She seemed to be in the middle of some eager speech. What Anne first heard was—

"And so, I made her go. I could not bear that she should be frightened from the visit by such nonsense. What!—would I be turned back from doing a thing that I had determined to do, and that I knew to be right, by the airs and interference of such a person?—or of any person I may say. No,—I have no idea of being so easily persuaded. When I have made up my mind, I have made it. And Henrietta seemed entirely to have made up hers to call at Winthrop to-day—and yet, she was as near giving it up, out of nonsensical complaisance!"

"She would have turned back then, but for you?"

"She would indeed. I am almost ashamed to say it."

"Happy for her, to have such a mind as yours at hand! After the hints you gave just now, which did but confirm my own observations, the last time I was in company with him, I need not affect to have no comprehension of what is going on. I see that more than a mere dutiful morning visit to your aunt was in question;—and woe betide him, and her too, when it comes to things of consequence, when they are placed in circumstances, requiring fortitude and strength of mind, if she have not resolution enough to resist idle interference in such a trifle as this. Your sister is an amiable creature; but *yours* is the character of decision and firmness, I see. If you value her conduct or happiness, infuse as much of your own spirit into her, as you can. But this, no doubt, you have been always doing. It is the worst evil of too yielding and indecisive a character, that no influence over it can be depended on. —You are never sure of a good impression being durable. Every body may sway it. Let those who would be happy be firm. Here is a nut," said he, catching one down from an upper bough. "to exemplify,—a beautiful glossy nut, which, blessed with original strength, has outlived all the storms of autumn. Not a puncture, not a weak spot any where. This nut," he continued, with playful solemnity,—"while so many of his brethren have fallen and been trodden under foot, is still in possession of all the happiness that a hazel-nut can be supposed capable of." Then returning to his former earnest tone: "My first wish, for all whom I am interested in, is that they should be firm. If Louisa Musgrove would be beautiful and happy in her November of life, she will cherish all her present powers of mind."

He had done,—and was unanswered. It would have surprised Anne if Louisa could have readily answered such a speech—words of such interest, spoken with such serious warmth!—she could imagine what Louisa was feeling. For herself—she feared to move, lest she should be seen. While she remained, a bush of low rambling holly protected her, and they were moving on. Before they were beyond her hearing, however, Louisa spoke again.

"Mary is good-natured enough in many respects," said she; "but she does sometimes provoke me excessively, by her nonsense and pride; the Elliot pride. She has a great deal too much of the Elliot pride. —We do so wish that Charles had married Anne instead. —I suppose you know he wanted to marry Anne?"

After a moment's pause, Captain Wentworth said—

"Do you mean that she refused him?"

"Oh! yes, certainly."

"When did that happen?"

"I do not exactly know, for Henrietta and I were at school at the time; but I believe about a year before he married Mary. I wish she had accepted him. We should all have liked her a great deal better; and papa and mamma always think it was her great friend Lady Russell's doing, that she did not. —They think Charles might not be learned and bookish enough to please Lady Russell, and that therefore, she persuaded Anne to refuse him."

The sounds were retreating, and Anne distinguished no more. Her own emotions still kept her fixed. She had much to recover from, before she could move. The listener's proverbial fate was not absolutely hers; she had heard no evil of herself—but she had heard a great deal of very painful import. She saw how her own character was considered by Captain Wentworth; and there had been just that degree of feeling and curiosity about her in his manner which must give her extreme agitation.

As soon as she could, she went after Mary, and having found, and walked back with her to their former station, by the stile, felt some comfort in their whole party being immediately afterwards collected, and once more in motion together. Her spirits wanted the solitude and silence which only numbers could give.

Charles and Henrietta returned, bringing, as may be conjectured, Charles Hayter with them. The minutiæ of the business Anne could not attempt to understand; even Captain Wentworth did not seem admitted to perfect confidence here; but that there had been a withdrawing on the gentleman's side, and a relenting on the lady's, and that they were now very glad to be together again, did not admit a doubt. Henrietta looked a little ashamed, but very well pleased;—Charles Hayter exceedingly happy, and they were devoted to each other almost from the first instant of their all setting forward for Uppercross.

Everything now marked out Louisa for Captain Wentworth; nothing could be plainer; and where many divisions were necessary, or even where they were not, they walked side by side, nearly as much as the other two. In a long strip of meadow-land, where there was ample space for all, they were thus divided— forming three distinct parties; and to that party of the three which boasted least animation, and least complaisance, Anne necessarily belonged. She joined Charles and Mary, and was tired enough to be very glad of Charles's other arm;—but Charles, though in very good humour with her, was out of temper with his wife. Mary had shewn herself disobliging to him, and was now to reap the consequence, which consequence was his dropping her arm almost every moment to cut off the heads of some nettles in the hedge with his switch; and when Mary began to complain of it, and lament her being ill-used, according to custom, in being on the hedge side, while Anne was never incommoded on the other, he dropped the arms of both to hunt after a weasel which he had a momentary glance of, and they could hardly get him along at all.

This long meadow bordered a lane, which their footpath, at the end of it was to cross; and when the party had all reached the gate of exit, the carriage advancing in the same direction, which had been some time heard, was just coming up, and proved to be Admiral Croft's gig. —He and his wife had taken their intended drive, and were returning home. Upon hearing how long a walk the young people had engaged in, they kindly offered a seat to any lady who might be particularly tired; it would save her a full mile, and they were going through Uppercross. The invitation was general, and generally declined. The Miss Musgroves were not at all tired, and Mary was either offended, by not being asked before any of the others, or what Louisa called the Elliot pride could not endure to make a third in a one horse chaise.

The walking-party had crossed the lane, and were surmounting an opposite stile; and the admiral was putting his horse in motion again, when Captain Wentworth cleared the hedge in a moment to say something to his sister. —The something might be guessed by its effects.

"Miss Elliot, I am sure *you* are tired," cried Mrs Croft. "Do let us have the pleasure of taking you home. Here is excellent room for three, I assure you. If we were all like you, I believe we might sit four. —You must, indeed, you must."

Anne was still in the lane; and though instinctively beginning to decline, she was not allowed to proceed. The Admiral's kind urgency came in support of his wife's; they would not be refused; they compressed themselves into the smallest possible space to leave her a corner, and Captain Wentworth, without saying a word, turned to her, and quietly obliged her to be assisted into the carriage.

Yes,—he had done it. She was in the carriage, and felt that he had placed her there, that his will and his hands had done it, that she owed it to his perception of her fatigue, and his resolution to give her rest. She was very much affected by the view of his disposition towards her which all these things made apparent. This little circumstance seemed the completion of all that had gone before. She understood him. He could not forgive her,—but he could not be unfeeling. Though condemning her for the past, and considering it with high and unjust resentment, though perfectly careless of her, and though becoming attached to another, still he could not see her suffer, without the desire of giving her relief. It was a remainder of former sentiment; it was an impulse of pure, though unacknowledged friendship; it was a proof of his own warm and amiable heart, which she could not contemplate without emotions so compounded of pleasure and pain, that she knew not which prevailed.

Plato
FROM PHAEDRUS

Translated by Benjamin Jowett

Persons of the Dialogue: Socrates; Phaedrus.
Scene: Under a plane-tree, by the banks of the Ilissus.

SOCRATES: My dear Phaedrus, whence come you, and whither are you going?

PHAEDRUS: I come from Lysias the son of Cephalus, and I am going to take a walk outside the wall, for I have been sitting with him the whole morning; and our common friend Acumenus tells me that it is much more refreshing to walk in the open air than to be shut up in a cloister.

SOCRATES: There he is right. Lysias then, I suppose, was in the town?

PHAEDRUS: Yes, he was staying with Epicrates, here at the house of Morychus; that house which is near the temple of Olympian Zeus.

SOCRATES: And how did he entertain you? Can I be wrong in supposing that Lysias gave you a feast of discourse?

PHAEDRUS: You shall hear, if you can spare time to accompany me.

SOCRATES: And should I not deem the conversation of you and Lysias "a thing of higher import," as I may say in the words of Pindar, "than any business"?

PHAEDRUS: Will you go on?

SOCRATES: And will you go on with the narration?

PHAEDRUS: My tale, Socrates, is one of your sort, for love was the theme which occupied us—love after a fashion: Lysias has been writing about a fair youth who was being tempted, but not by a lover; and this was the point: he ingeniously proved that the non-lover should be accepted rather than the lover.

SOCRATES: O that is noble of him! I wish that he would say the poor man rather than the rich, and the old man rather than the young one; then he would meet the case of me and of many a man; his words would be quite refreshing, and he would be a public benefactor. For my part, I do so long to hear his speech, that if you walk all the way to Megara, and when you have reached the wall come back, as Herodicus recommends, without going in, I will keep you company.

PHAEDRUS: What do you mean, my good Socrates? How can you imagine that my unpractised memory can do justice to an elaborate work, which the greatest rhetorician of the age spent a long time in composing. Indeed, I cannot; I would give a great deal if I could.

SOCRATES: I believe that I know Phaedrus about as well as I know myself, and I am very sure that the speech of Lysias was repeated to him, not once only, but again and again;—he insisted on hearing it many times over and Lysias was very willing to gratify him; at last, when nothing else would do, he got hold of the book, and looked at what he most wanted to see,—this occupied him during the whole morning; —and then when he was tired with sitting, he went out to take a walk, not until, by the dog, as I believe, he had simply learned by heart the entire discourse, unless it was unusually long, and he went to a place outside the wall that he might practise his lesson. There he saw a certain lover of discourse who had a similar weakness;—he saw and rejoiced; now thought he, "I shall have a partner in my revels." And he invited him to come and walk with him. But when the lover of discourse begged that he would repeat the tale, he gave himself airs and said, "No I cannot," as if he were indisposed; although, if the hearer had refused, he would sooner or later have been compelled by him to listen whether he would or no. Therefore,

Phaedrus, bid him do at once what he will soon do whether bidden or not.

PHAEDRUS: I see that you will not let me off until I speak in some fashion or other; verily therefore my best plan is to speak as I best can.

SOCRATES: A very true remark, that of yours.

PHAEDRUS: I will do as I say; but believe me, Socrates, I did not learn the very words—O no; nevertheless I have a general notion of what he said, and will give you a summary of the points in which the lover differed from the non-lover. Let me begin at the beginning.

SOCRATES: Yes, my sweet one; but you must first of all show what you have in your left hand under your cloak, for that roll, as I suspect, is the actual discourse. Now, much as I love you, I would not have you suppose that I am going to have your memory exercised at my expense, if you have Lysias himself here.

PHAEDRUS: Enough; I see that I have no hope of practising my art upon you. But if I am to read, where would you please to sit?

SOCRATES: Let us turn aside and go by the Ilissus; we will sit down at some quiet spot.

PHAEDRUS: I am fortunate in not having my sandals, and as you never have any, I think that we may go along the brook and cool our feet in the water; this will be the easiest way, and at midday and in the summer is far from being unpleasant.

SOCRATES: Lead on, and look out for a place in which we can sit down.

PHAEDRUS: Do you see the tallest plane-tree in the distance?

SOCRATES: Yes.

PHAEDRUS: There are shade and gentle breezes, and grass on which we may either sit or lie down.

SOCRATES: Move forward.

PHAEDRUS: I should like to know, Socrates, whether the place is not somewhere here at which Boreas is said to have carried off Orithyia from the banks of the Ilissus?

SOCRATES: Such is the tradition.

PHAEDRUS: And is this the exact spot? The little stream is delightfully clear and bright; I can fancy that there might be maidens playing near.

SOCRATES: I believe that the spot is not exactly here, but about a quarter of a mile lower down, where you cross to the temple of Artemis, and there is, I think, some sort of an altar of Boreas at the place.

PHAEDRUS: I have never noticed it; but I beseech you to tell me, Socrates, do you believe this tale?

SOCRATES: The wise are doubtful, and I should not be singular if, like them, I too doubted. I might have a rational explanation that Orithyia was playing with Pharmacia, when a northern gust carried her over the neighbouring rocks; and this being the manner of her death, she was said to have been carried away by Boreas. There is a discrepancy, however, about the locality; according to another version of the story she was taken from Areopagus, and not from this place. Now I quite acknowledge that these allegories are very nice, but he is not to be envied who has to invent them; much labour and ingenuity will be required of him; and when he has once begun, he must go on and rehabilitate Hippocentaurs and chimeras dire. Gorgons and winged steeds flow in apace, and numberless other inconceivable and portentous natures. And if he is sceptical about them, and would fain reduce them one after another to the rules of probability, this sort of crude philosophy will take up a great deal of time. Now I have no leisure for such enquiries; shall I tell you why? I must first know myself, as the Delphian inscription says; to be curious about that which is not my concern, while I am still in ignorance of my own self, would be ridiculous. And therefore I bid farewell to all this; the common opinion is enough for me. For, as I was saying, I want to know not about this, but about myself: am I a monster more complicated and swollen with passion than the serpent Typho, or a creature of a gentler and simpler sort, to whom Nature has given a diviner and lowlier destiny? But let me ask you, friend: have we not reached the plane-tree to which you were conducting us?

PHAEDRUS: Yes, this is the tree.

SOCRATES: By Herè, a fair resting-place, full of summer sounds and scents. Here is this lofty and spreading plane-tree, and the agnus cast us high and clustering, in the fullest blossom and the greatest fragrance; and the stream which flows beneath the plane-tree is deliciously cold to the feet. Judging from the ornaments and images, this must be a spot sacred to Achelous and the Nymphs. How delightful is the breeze: —so very sweet; and there is a sound in the air shrill and summerlike which makes answer to the chorus of the cicadae. But the greatest charm of all is the grass, like a pillow gently sloping to the head. My dear Phaedrus, you have been an admirable guide.

PHAEDRUS: What an incomprehensible being you are, Socrates: when you are in the country, as you say, you really are like some stranger who is led about by a guide. Do you ever cross the border? I rather think that you never venture even outside the gates.

SOCRATES: Very true, my good friend; and I hope that you will excuse me when you hear the reason, which is, that I am a lover of knowledge, and the men who dwell in the city are my teachers, and not the trees or the country. Though I do indeed believe that you have found a spell with which to draw me out of the city into the country, like a hungry cow before whom a bough or a bunch of fruit is waved. For only hold up before me in like manner a book, and you may lead me all round Attica, and over the wide world. And now having arrived, I intend to lie down, and do you choose any posture in which you can read best. Begin.

William Wordsworth
FROM THE PRELUDE (1805)

Those walks did now, like a returning spring,
Come back on me again. When first I made
Once more the circuit of our little Lake
If ever happiness hath lodg'd with man,
That day consummate happiness was mine,
Wide-spreading, steady, calm, contemplative.
The sun was set, or setting, when I left
Our cottage door, and evening soon brought on
A sober hour, not winning or serene,
For cold and raw the air was, and untun'd:
But, as a face we love is sweetest then
When sorrow damps it, or, whatever look
It chance to wear is sweetest if the heart
Have fulness in itself, even so with me
It fared that evening. Gently did my soul
Put off her veil, and, self-transmuted, stood
Naked as in the presence of her God.
As on I walked, a comfort seem'd to touch
A heart that had not been disconsolate,
Strength came where weakness was not known to be,
At least not felt; and restoration came,
Like an intruder, knocking at the door
Of unacknowledg'd weariness.

Henry Vaughan
REGENERATION

1

A ward, and still in bonds, one day
   I stole abroad,
It was high-spring, and all the way
   Primros'd, and hung with shade;
   Yet, was it frost within,
    And surly winds
Blasted my infant buds, and sin
   Like Clouds eclips'd my mind.

2

Storm'd thus; I straight perceiv'd my spring
   Mere stage, and show,
My walk a monstrous, mountain'd thing
   Rough-cast with Rocks, and snow;
   And as a Pilgrims Eye
    Far from relief,
Measures the melancholy sky
   Then drops, and rains for grief,

3

So sigh'd I upwards still, at last
   'Twixt steps, and falls
I reach'd the pinacle, where plac'd
   I found a pair of scales,
   I took them up and laid
    In th' one late paines,
The other smoke, and pleasures weigh'd
   But prov'd the heavier grains;

4

With that, some cried, *Away;* straight I
　　Obey'd, and led
Full East, a fair, fresh field could spy
　　Some call'd it, *Jacobs Bed;*
　　A Virgin-soil, which no
　　Rude feet ere trod,
Where (since he stept there,) only go
　　Prophets, and friends of God.

5

Here, I repos'd; but scarce well set,
　　A grove descried
Of stately height, whose branches met
　　And mixt on every side;
　　I entered, and once in
　　(Amaz'd to see't,)
Found all was chang'd, and a new spring
　　Did all my senses greet;

6

The unthrift Sun shot vital gold
　　A thousand pieces,
And heaven its azure did unfold
　　Checqur'd with snowy fleeces,
　　The aire was all in spice
　　And every bush
A garland wore; Thus fed my Eyes
　　But all the Ear lay hush.

7

Only a little Fountain lent
　　Some use for Ears,
And on the dumb shades language spent
　　The Music of her tears;
　　I drew her near, and found

The Cistern full
Of divers stones, some bright, and round
    Others ill-shap'd, and dull.

8

The first (pray mark,) as quick as light
    Danc'd through the flood,
But, th' last more heavy then the night
    Nail'd to the Center stood;
    I wonder'd much, but tired
        At last with thought,
My restless Eye that still desir'd
    As strange an object brought;

9

It was a bank of flowers, where I descried
    (Though 'twas mid-day,)
Some fast asleep, others broad-eyed
    And taking in the Ray,
    Here musing long, I heard
        A rushing wind
Which still increas'd, but whence it stirr'd
    No where I could not find;

10

I turn'd me round, and to each shade
    Dispatch'd an Eye,
To see, if any leaf had made
    Least motion, or Reply,
    But while I listning sought
        My mind to ease
By knowing, where 'twas, or where not,
    It whisper'd; *Where I please.*

Lord, then said I, *On me one breath,*
And let me die before my death!

William Wordsworth
RESOLUTION AND INDEPENDENCE

There was a roaring in the wind all night;
The rain came heavily and fell in floods;
But now the sun is rising calm and bright;
The birds are singing in the distant woods;
Over his own sweet voice the Stock-dove broods;
The Jay makes answer as the Magpie chatters;
And all the air is filled with pleasant noise of waters.

All things that love the sun are out of doors;
The sky rejoices in the morning's birth;
The grass is bright with rain-drops;—on the moors
The hare is running races in her mirth;
And with her feet she from the plashy earth
Raises a mist; that, glittering in the sun,
Runs with her all the way, wherever she doth run.

I was a Traveller then upon the moor;
I saw the hare that raced about with joy;
I heard the woods and distant waters roar;
Or heard them not, as happy as a boy:
The pleasant season did my heart employ:
My old remembrances went from me wholly;
And all the ways of men, so vain and melancholy.

But, as it sometimes chanceth, from the might
Of joys in minds that can no further go,
As high as we have mounted in delight
In our dejection do we sink as low;
To me that morning did it happen so;

And fears and fancies thick upon me came;
Dim sadness—and blind thoughts, I knew not, nor could name.

I heard the sky-lark warbling in the sky;
And I bethought me of the playful hare:
Even such a happy Child of earth am I;
Even as these blissful creatures do I fare;
Far from the world I walk, and from all care;
But there may come another day to me—
Solitude, pain of heart, distress, and poverty.

My whole life I have lived in pleasant thought,
As if life's business were a summer mood;
As if all needful things would come unsought
To genial faith, still rich in genial good;
But how can He expect that others should
Build for him, sow for him, and at his call
Love him, who for himself will take no heed at all?

I thought of Chatterton, the marvellous Boy,
The sleepless Soul that perished in his pride;
Of Him who walked in glory and in joy
Following his plough, along the mountain-side:
By our own spirits are we deified:
We Poets in our youth begin in gladness;
But thereof come in the end despondency and madness.

Now, whether it were by peculiar grace,
A leading from above, a something given,
Yet it befell, that, in this lonely place,
When I with these untoward thoughts had striven,
Beside a pool bare to the eye of heaven
I saw a Man before me unawares:
The oldest man he seemed that ever wore grey hairs.

As a huge stone is sometimes seen to lie
Couched on the bald top of an eminence;
Wonder to all who do the same espy,
By what means it could thither come, and whence;
So that it seems a thing endued with sense:
Like a sea-beast crawled forth, that on a shelf
Of rock or sand reposeth, there to sun itself;

Such seemed this Man, not all alive nor dead,
Nor all asleep—in his extreme old age:
His body was bent double, feet and head
Coming together in life's pilgrimage;
As if some dire constraint of pain, or rage
Of sickness felt by him in times long past,
A more than human weight upon his frame had cast.

Himself he propped, limbs, body, and pale face,
Upon a long grey staff of shaven wood:
And, still as I drew near with gentle pace,
Upon the margin of that moorish flood
Motionless as a cloud the old Man stood,
That heareth not the loud winds when they call,
And moveth all together, if it move at all.

At length, himself unsettling, he the pond
Stirred with his staff, and fixedly did look
Upon the muddy water, which he conned,
As if he had been reading in a book:
And now a stranger's privilege I took;
And, drawing to his side, to him did say,
"This morning gives us promise of a glorious day."

A gentle answer did the old Man make,
In courteous speech which forth he slowly drew:
And him with further words I thus bespake,

"What occupation do you there pursue?
This is a lonesome place for one like you."
Ere he replied, a flash of mild surprise
Broke from the sable orbs of his yet-vivid eyes.

His words came feebly, from a feeble chest,
But each in solemn order followed each,
With something of a lofty utterance drest—
Choice word and measured phrase, above the reach
Of ordinary men; a stately speech;
Such as grave Livers do in Scotland use,
Religious men, who give to God and man their dues.

He told, that to these waters he had come
To gather leeches, being old and poor:
Employment hazardous and wearisome!
And he had many hardships to endure:
From pond to pond he roamed, from moor to moor;
Housing, with God's good help, by choice or chance;
And in this way he gained an honest maintenance.

The old Man still stood talking by my side;
But now his voice to me was like a stream
Scarce heard; nor word from word could I divide;
And the whole body of the Man did seem
Like one whom I had met with in a dream;
Or like a man from some far region sent,
To give me human strength, by apt admonishment.

My former thoughts returned: the fear that kills;
And hope that is unwilling to be fed;
Cold, pain, and labour, and all fleshly ills;
And mighty Poets in their misery dead.
—Perplexed, and longing to be comforted,
My question eagerly did I renew,

"How is it that you live, and what is it you do?"

He with a smile did then his words repeat;
And said that, gathering leeches, far and wide
He travelled; stirring thus about his feet
The waters of the pools where they abide.
"Once I could meet with them on every side;
But they have dwindled long by slow decay;
Yet still I persevere, and find them where I may."

While he was talking thus, the lonely place,
The old Man's shape, and speech—all troubled me:
In my mind's eye I seemed to see him pace
About the weary moors continually,
Wandering about alone and silently.
While I these thoughts within myself pursued,
He, having made a pause, the same discourse renewed.

And soon with this he other matter blended,
Cheerfully uttered, with demeanour kind,
But stately in the main; and, when he ended,
I could have laughed myself to scorn to find
In that decrepit Man so firm a mind.
"God," said I, "be my help and stay secure;
I'll think of the Leech-gatherer on the lonely moor!"

Wendell Berry
RETURNING

I was walking in a dark valley
and above me the tops of the hills
had caught the morning light.
I heard the light singing as it went out
among the grassblades and the leaves.
I waded upward through the shadow
until my head emerged,
my shoulders were mantled with the light,
and my whole body came up
out of the darkness, and stood
on the new shore of the day.
Where I had come was home,
for my own house stood white
where the dark river wore the earth.
The sheen of bounty was on the grass,
and the spring of the year had come.

Jean-Jacques Rousseau
FROM THE REVERIES OF A SOLITARY WALKER

SECOND WALK

Having, then, formed the project of describing the habitual state of my soul in the strongest position in which a mortal could ever find himself, I saw no simpler and surer way to carry out this enterprise than to keep a faithful record of my solitary walks and of the reveries which fill them when I leave my head entirely free and let my ideas follow their bent without resistance or constraint. These hours of solitude and meditation are the only ones in the day during which I am fully myself and for myself, without diversion, without obstacle, and during which I can truly claim to be what nature willed.

I soon felt I had too long delayed carrying out this project. Already less lively, my imagination no longer bursts into flame the way it used to in contemplating the object which stimulates it. I delight less in the delirium of reverie. Henceforth there is more reminiscence than creation in what it produces. A tepid languor enervates all my faculties. The spirit of life is gradually dying out in me. Only with difficulty does my soul any longer thrust itself out of its decrepit wrapping; and were it not that I am hopeful of reaching the state to which I aspire because I feel I have a right to it, I would no longer exist but by memories. Thus, in order to contemplate myself before my decline, I must go back at least a few years to the time when, losing all hope here-below and no longer finding any food here on earth for my heart, I gradually became accustomed to feeding it with its own substance and to looking within myself for all its nourishment.

This resource, which I thought of too late, became so fruitful that it soon sufficed to compensate for everything. The habit of turning within eventually made me stop feeling and almost stop remembering my ills. By my own experience, I thus learned that the source of true happiness is within us and that it is not within the power of men to make anyone who can will to be happy truly miserable. For four or five years, I habitually tasted those internal delights that loving and sweet souls find in contemplation. Those moments of rapture, those ecstasies, which I sometimes experienced in walking around alone that way, were enjoyments I owed to my persecutors. Without them I would never have found or become cognizant of the treasures I carried within myself. In the midst of so many riches, how could a faithful record of them be kept? In wanting to recall so many sweet reveries, instead of describing them, I fell back into them. This is a state which is brought back by being remembered and of which we would soon cease to be aware, if we completely ceased feeling it.

I fully experienced this effect during the walks which followed my plans to write the sequel to my *Confessions,* especially during the one I am going to speak of and during which an unforeseen accident came to interrupt the thread of my ideas and give them another direction for some time.

After lunch on Thursday, the 24th of October, 1776, I followed the boulevards as far as the Rue du Chemin-Vert which I took up to the heights of Ménilmontant and from there, taking paths across the vineyards and meadows as far as Charonne, I crossed over the cheerful countryside which separates these two villages; then I made a detour in order to come back across the same meadows by taking a different route. In wandering over them, I enjoyed that pleasure and interest which charming places have always given me and stopped from time to time to look at plants in the vegetation. I noticed two I quite rarely saw around Paris, but which I found to be very abundant in that area. One is the *Picris hieracioides,* belonging to the family of composite plants; and the other is the *Buplevrum falcatum,* belonging to the family of umbelliferous plants. This discovery delighted and amused me for a very long time and ended in the discovery of an even rarer plant, especially in high places, namely, the *Cerastium aquaticum* which, in spite of the accident that befell me the same day, I have come across in a book I had with me and have now placed in my herbarium.

Finally, after having looked thoroughly at several other plants I saw still in bloom and which I was always pleased to see even though I was familiar with their aspect and name, I gradually turned away from these minute observations so as to give myself up to the no less charming, but more moving, impression which the whole scene made on me. A few days before, the grape-gathering had been completed; strollers from the city had already withdrawn;

even the peasants were leaving the fields until the toils of winter. The countryside, still green and cheerful, but partly defoliated and already almost desolate, presented everywhere an image of solitude and of winter's approach. Its appearance gave rise to a mixed impression, sweet and sad, too analogous to my age and lot for me not to make the connection. I saw myself at the decline of an innocent and unfortunate life, my soul still full of vivacious feelings and my mind still bedecked with a few flowers—but flowers already wilted by sadness and dried up by worries. Alone and forsaken, I felt the coming cold of the first frosts, and my flagging imagination no longer filled my solitude with beings formed according to my heart. Sighing, I said to myself: "What have I done here-below? I was made to live, and I am dying without having lived. At least it has not been my fault; and I will carry to the author of my being, if not an offering of good works which I have not been permitted to perform, at least a tribute of frustrated good intentions, of healthy feelings rendered ineffectual, and of a patience impervious to the scorn of men." I was moved by these reflections; I went back over the movements of my soul from the time of my youth, through my mature age, since having been sequestered from the society of men, and during the long seclusion in which I must finish my days. I mulled over all the affections of my heart with satisfaction, over its so tender but blind attachements, over the less sad than consoling ideas on which my mind had nourished itself for some years; and with a pleasure almost equal to that I had in giving myself up to this musing, I prepared to remember them well enough to describe them. My afternoon was spent in these peaceful meditations, and I was coming back very satisfied with my day when, at the height of my reverie, I was dragged out of it by the event which remains for me to relate.

I was on the road down from Ménilmontant almost opposite the Galant Jardinier at about six o'clock when some people walking ahead of me suddenly swerved aside and I saw a huge Great Dane rushing down upon me. Racing before a carriage, the dog had no time to check its pace or to turn aside when it noticed me. I judged that the only means I had to avoid being knocked to the ground was to make a great leap, so well-timed that the dog would pass under me while I was still in the air. This idea, quicker than a flash and which I had the time neither to think through nor carry out, was my last before my accident. I did not feel the blow, nor the fall, nor anything of what followed until the moment I came to.

It was almost night when I regained consciousness. I found myself in the arms of three or four young people who told me what had just happened to me. The Great Dane, unable to check its bound, had collided against my legs and, bowling me over with its mass and speed, had caused me to fall head first: my upper jaw had struck against a very rough pavement with the whole weight of my body behind it; and the shock of the fall was even greater because I was walking downhill and my head had struck lower than my feet.

The carriage the dog was with was following right behind it and would have run me over had the coachman not reined in his horses instantly. That is what I learned from the account of those who had picked me up and who were still holding me up when I came to. The state in which I found myself in that instant is too unusual not to give a description of here.

Night was coming on. I perceived the sky, some stars, and a little greenery. This first sensation was a delicious moment. I still had no feeling of myself except as being "over there." I was born into life at that instant, and it seemed to me that I filled all the objects I perceived with my frail existence. Entirely absorbed in the present moment, I remembered nothing; I had no distinct notion of my person nor the least idea of what had just happened to me; I knew neither who I was nor where I was; I felt neither injury, fear, nor worry. I watched my blood flow as I would have watched a brook flow, without even suspecting that this blood belonged to me in any way. I felt a rapturous calm in my whole being; and each time I remember it, I find nothing comparable to it in all the activity of known pleasures.

They asked me where I lived; it was impossible for me to say. I asked where I was: they told me: "at the Haute-Borne." They might just as well have said: "on Mount Atlas." In succession, I had to ask what country I found myself in, what city, and what district. Even that was not enough for me to know where I was. It took me the whole distance from there to the boulevard to recall my address and my name. A gentleman I did not know, but who was charitable enough to accompany me a little way, learning that I lived so far away, counseled me to get a cab at the Temple to take me home. I walked easily and sprightly, feeling neither pain nor hurt, although I kept spitting out a lot of blood. But I had an icy shiver which made my jarred teeth chatter in a very uncomfortable way. When I reached the Temple, I thought that since I was walking without trouble it was better to continue on foot than to risk perishing from cold in a cab. Thus I covered the half-league from the Temple to the Rue Platrière, walking without trouble, avoiding obstacles and coaches, choosing and following my way just as well as I would have done in perfect health. I arrived, opened the lock they had installed at the street door, climbed the staircase in darkness, and finally entered my home without incident, apart from my fall and its consequences, of which, even then, I was not yet fully aware.

My wife's cries upon seeing me made me understand that I was worse off than I thought. I passed the night without yet being aware of, or feeling, my injuries. Here is what I felt and discovered the next day: my upper lip was split on the inside up to my nose; outside, the skin had held firm and prevented the lip from being split completely open; four teeth had been pushed into my upper jaw; the whole part of the face which covers it was extremely swollen and skinned; my right thumb was sprained and very large; my left thumb hurt painfully; my left arm was sprained; my left knee was also very swollen, and a severely painful bruise totally prevented me from bending it. But with all this upset, nothing broken, not even a tooth: now in a fall like this one, that is good luck bordering on the marvelous.

That, very faithfully, is the story of my accident. In a few days this story spread through Paris, so changed and distorted that it was impossible to recognize it in any way. I should have counted on this metamorphosis in advance. But so many bizarre circumstances were joined to it, so many obscure remarks and reticences accompanied it, they spoke to me about it in such a ridiculously discreet manner, that all these mysteries worried me. I have always hated the dark; it naturally fills me with a dread which the darkness they have surrounded me with for so many years could not have diminished. Of all the unusual events of this time period, I will relate only one, but one sufficient to permit judgment about the others.

M. Lenoir, lieutenant general of the police, with whom I had never had any dealings, sent his secretary to inquire about my tidings and to tender me pressing offers of service which, given the circumstances, appeared to me to be of no great use for my relief. His secretary did not fail to urge me very insistently to avail myself of these offers, even going so far as to tell me that if I did not trust him, I could write directly to M. Lenoir. This great eagerness and the confidential manner which accompanied it led me to understand that beneath it all was some mystery which I tried in vain to penetrate. Hardly that much was needed to alarm me, especially given the state of agitation my head was in from my accident and the resultant fever. I abandoned myself to a thousand troubling and sad conjectures and made commentaries on everything which went on around me, commentaries which were more a sign of the delirium of fever than of the composure of a man who no longer takes interest in anything.

Another event occurred which completely destroyed my serenity. Mme d'Ormoy had sought me out for some years without my having been able to guess why. Pretentious little gifts and frequent visits without purpose or pleasure showed me well enough that she had a secret goal in all that, but not well enough what that goal was. She had spoken to me of a novel she wanted to write to present to the queen. I had told her what I thought of women authors. She had intimated that the goal of this project was to restore her fortunes, a goal for which she needed protection; I had nothing to reply to that. She later told me that, having been unable to gain access to the queen, she was determined to give her book to the public. It was no longer the moment to give her advice she had not asked me for and which she would not have followed. She had spoken of showing me the manuscript beforehand. I begged her to do nothing of the sort, and she did nothing of the sort.

One fine day during my convalescence I received this book from her completely printed and even bound. In the preface I saw such swollen praises of me, laid on so clumsily and with so much affectation, that I was disagreeably impressed by them. The crude fawning which was so perceptible in it was never associated with benevolence; about that, my heart could never be deceived.

A few days later, Mme d'Ormoy and her daughter came to see me. She informed me that because of a note it contained, her book was causing the greatest fuss. I had hardly noticed this note while flipping rapidly through the novel. I reread the note after Mme d'Ormoy's departure. I examined the way it was constructed. I believed that in it I discovered the motive for her visits, her wheedlings, and the swollen praises of her preface; and I judged that there was no other goal in all of this than to dispose the public to attribute the note to me and consequently to burden me with the blame it would attract to its author in the circumstances under which it was published.

I had no means of putting an end to this fuss and the impression it could make; the only thing I could do was not foster it by continuing to endure the vain and ostensive visits of Mme d'Ormoy and her daughter. Here is the note I wrote to the mother for this purpose:

"Rousseau, not receiving any authors in his home, thanks Mme d'Ormoy for her kindness and begs her to honor him with her visits no more."

She replied to me by a letter, honest in appearance but contrived, like all those which people write to me in such cases. I had barbarously plunged a dagger into her sensitive heart and I must believe by the tone of her letter that because of her intense and true feelings for me, she would never endure this break without dying. So it is that straightforwardness and frankness in everything are horrid crimes in the world, and I appear nasty and ferocious to my contemporaries when I am guilty of no other crime in their eyes than that of not being false and perfidious as they.

I had already gone outside several times and had even strolled in the Tuileries quite a few times when I saw, by the astonishment of several of those who met me, that there was still another bit of news concerning me of which I was ignorant. I finally learned that it was rumored that I had died from my fall; and this rumor spread so rapidly and so obstinately that, more than two weeks after I had become aware of it, the king himself and the queen spoke of it as of something certain. In announcing this happy bit of news the *Avignon Courier,* according to what someone had the concern to write me, did not fail on this occasion to give a preview of the tribute of outrages and indignities which are being prepared in the form of a funeral oration in memory of me after my death.

This news was accompanied by an even more unusual circumstance which I learned of only by chance and which I have not been able to learn about in any detail. It is that they had at the same time started a subscription for printing the manuscripts they would find in my home. By that I understood that they were keeping a collection of fabricated writings available just for the purpose of attributing them to me right after my death: for to think they would faithfully print any of those they would actually find is a folly that cannot enter into the mind of a sensible man and from which fifteen years of experience have only too well protected me.

These observations, made one after the other and followed by many others which were scarcely less astonishing, caused my imagination, which I had believed to be calmed down, to become alarmed all over again, And this black darkness with which they relentlessly surrounded me rekindled all the dread it naturally inspires in me. I wore myself out making a thousand commentaries on it all and trying to understand the mysteries they rendered inexplicable for me. The only constant result of so many enigmas was to confirm all of my previous conclusions, to wit, that my personal fate and that of my reputation have been so fastened by the connivance of the whole present generation that no effort on my part could free me, since it is completely impossible for me to transmit any bequest to other ages without making it pass in this age through the hands of those interested in suppressing it.

But this time, I went further. The accumulation of so many fortuitous circumstances, the elevation of all of my cruelest enemies favored, so to speak, by fortune; all those who govern the state, all those who direct public opinion, all the people in official positions, all the men of influence, picked and culled as it were from among those who have some secret animosity against me in order to concur in the common plot; this universal agreement is too extraordinary to be purely fortuitous. If there had been a single man who had refused to be an accomplice to it, a single event which had gone against it, a single unforeseen circumstance which had been an obstacle to it, any of that would have been enough to make it fail. But all the acts of will, all the unlucky events, fortune and all its revolutions have made firm the work of men. And such a striking concurrence, which borders on the prodigious, cannot let me doubt that its complete success is written among the eternal decrees. Swarms of individual observations, either in the past or in the present, so confirm me in this opinion that I cannot prevent myself from henceforth considering as one of those secrets of Heaven impenetrable to human reason the same work that until now I looked upon as only a fruit of the wickedness of men.

This idea, far from being cruel and rending to me, consoles me, calms me, and helps me to resign myself. I do not go as far as St. Augustine who would have consoled himself to be damned if such had been the will of God. My resignation comes, it is true, from a less disinterested source, but one no less pure and to my mind, more worthy of the perfect Being whom I adore. God is just; He wills that I suffer; and He knows that I am innocent. That is the cause of my confidence; my heart and my reason cry out to me that I will not be deceived by it. Let me, therefore, leave men and fate to go their ways. Let me learn to suffer without a murmur. In the end, everything must return to order, and my turn will come, sooner or later.

Robert Frost
THE ROAD NOT TAKEN

Two roads diverged in a yellow wood,
And sorry I could not travel both
And be one traveler, long I stood
And looked down one as far as I could
To where it bent in the undergrowth;

Then took the other, as just as fair,
And having perhaps the better claim,
Because it was grassy and wanted wear;
Though as for that the passing there
Had worn them really about the same,

And both that morning equally lay
In leaves no step had trodden black.
Oh, I kept the first for another day!
Yet knowing how way leads on to way,
I doubted if I should ever come back.

I shall be telling this with a sigh
Somewhere ages and ages hence:
Two roads diverged in a wood, and I—
I took the one less traveled by,
And that has made all the difference.

Wendell Berry
SETTING OUT

for Gurney Norman

Even love must pass through loneliness,
the husbandman become again
the Long Hunter, and set out
not to the familiar woods of home,
but to the forest of the night,
the true wilderness, where renewal
is found, the lay of the ground
a premonition of the unknown.
Blowing leaf and flying wren
lead him on. He can no longer be at home,
he cannot return, unless he begin
the circle that first will carry him away.

Walt Whitman
SONG OF THE OPEN ROAD

1

Afoot and light-hearted I take to the open road,
Healthy, free, the world before me,
The long brown path before me leading wherever I choose.

Henceforth I ask not good-fortune, I myself am good-fortune,
Henceforth I whimper no more, postpone no more, need nothing,
Done with indoor complaints, libraries, querulous criticisms,
Strong and content I travel the open road.

The earth, that is sufficient,
I do not want the constellations any nearer,
I know they are very well where they are,
I know they suffice for those who belong to them.

(Still here I carry my old delicious burdens,
I carry them, men and women, I carry them with me wherever I go,
I swear it is impossible for me to get rid of them,
I am fill'd with them, and I will fill them in return.)

2

You road I enter upon and look around, I believe you are not all that is here,
I believe that much unseen is also here.

Here the profound lesson of reception, nor preference nor denial,
The black with his woolly head, the felon, the diseas'd, the illiterate person,
    are not denied;
The birth, the hasting after the physician, the beggar's tramp, the drunkard's
    stagger, the laughing party of mechanics,
The escaped youth, the rich person's carriage, the fop, the eloping couple,

The early market-man, the hearse, the moving of furniture into the town, the
    return back from the town,
They pass, I also pass, any thing passes, none can be interdicted,
None but are accepted, none but shall be dear to me.

3
You air that serves me with breath to speak!
You objects that call from diffusion my meanings and give them shape!
You light that wraps me and all things in delicate equable showers!
You paths worn in the irregular hollows by the roadsides!
I believe you are latent with unseen existences, you are so dear to me.

You flagg'd walks of the cities! you strong curbs at the edges!
You ferries! you planks and posts of wharves! you timber-lined sides! you distant
    ships!

You rows of houses! you window-pierc'd façades! you roofs!
You porches and entrances! you copings and iron guards!
You windows whose transparent shells might expose so much!
You doors and ascending steps! you arches!
You gray stones of interminable pavements! you trodden crossings!
From all that has touch'd you I believe you have imparted to yourselves, and
    now would impart the same secretly to me,
From the living and the dead you have peopled your impassive surfaces, and
    the spirits thereof would be evident and amicable with me.

4
The earth expanding right hand and left hand,
The picture alive, every part in its best light,
The music falling in where it is wanted, and stopping where it is not wanted,
The cheerful voice of the public road, the gay fresh sentiment of the road.

O highway I travel, do you say to me *Do not leave me?*
Do you say *Venture not—if you leave me you are lost?*
Do you say *I am already prepared, I am well-beaten and undenied, adhere to me?*

O public road, I say back I am not afraid to leave you, yet I love you,

You express me better than I can express myself,
You shall be more to me than my poem.

I think heroic deeds were all conceiv'd in the open air, and all free poems also,
I think I could stop here myself and do miracles,
I think whatever I shall meet on the road I shall like, and whoever beholds me
    shall like me,
I think whoever I see must be happy.

5

From this hour I ordain myself loos'd of limits and imaginary lines,
Going where I list, my own master total and absolute,
Listening to others, considering well what they say,
Pausing, searching, receiving, contemplating,
Gently, but with undeniable will, divesting myself of the holds that would hold
    me.
I inhale great draughts of space,
The east and the west are mine, and the north and the south are mine.

I am larger, better than I thought,
I did not know I held so much goodness.

All seems beautiful to me,
I can repeat over to men and women You have done such good to me I would
    do the same to you,
I will recruit for myself and you as I go,
I will scatter myself among men and women as I go,
I will toss a new gladness and roughness among them,
Whoever denies me it shall not trouble me,
Whoever accepts me he or she shall be blessed and shall bless me.

6

Now if a thousand perfect men were to appear it would not amaze me,

Now if a thousand beautiful forms of women appear'd it would not astonish me.

Now I see the secret of the making of the best persons,
It is to grow in the open air and to eat and sleep with the earth.

Here a great personal deed has room,
(Such a deed seizes upon the hearts of the whole race of men,
Its effusion of strength and will overwhelms law and mocks all
authority and all argument against it.)

Here is the test of wisdom,
Wisdom is not finally tested in schools,
Wisdom cannot be pass'd from one having it to another not having it,
Wisdom is of the soul, is not susceptible of proof, is its own proof,
Applies to all stages and objects and qualities and is content,
Is the certainty of the reality and immortality of things, and the excellence of
    things;
Something there is in the float of the sight of things that provokes it out of the
    soul.

Now I re-examine philosophies and religions,
They may prove well in lecture-rooms, yet not prove at all under the spacious
    clouds and along the landscape and flowing currents.

Here is realization,
Here is a man tallied—he realizes here what he has in him,
The past, the future, majesty, love—if they are vacant of you, you are vacant of
    them.

Only the kernel of every object nourishes;
Where is he who tears off the husks for you and me?
Where is he that undoes stratagems and envelopes for you and me?

Here is adhesiveness, it is not previously fashion'd, it is apropos;
Do you know what it is as you pass to be loved by strangers?
Do you know the talk of those turning eye-balls?

7

Here is the efflux of the soul,

The efflux of the soul comes from within through embower'd gates, ever provoking questions,

These yearnings why are they? these thoughts in the darkness why are they?

Why are there men and women that while they are nigh me the sunlight
  expands my blood?

Why when they leave me do my pennants of joy sink flat and lank?

Why are there trees I never walk under but large and melodious thoughts
  descend upon me?

(I think they hang there winter and summer on those trees and always drop
  fruit as I pass;)

What is it I interchange so suddenly with strangers?

What with some driver as I ride on the seat by his side?

What with some fisherman drawing his seine by the shore as I walk by and
  pause?

What gives me to be free to a woman's and man's good-will? what gives them
  to be free to mine?

8

The efflux of the soul is happiness, here is happiness,

I think it pervades the open air, waiting at all times,

Now it flows unto us, we are rightly charged.

Here rises the fluid and attaching character,

The fluid and attaching character is the freshness and sweetness of man and
  woman,

(The herbs of the morning sprout no fresher and sweeter every day out of the
  roots of themselves, than it sprouts fresh and sweet continually out of
  itself.)

Toward the fluid and attaching character exudes the sweat of the love of young
  and old,

From it falls distill'd the charm that mocks beauty and attainments,

Toward it heaves the shuddering longing ache of contact.

9

Allons! whoever you are come travel with me!
Traveling with me you find what never tires.

The earth never tires,
The earth is rude, silent, incomprehensible at first, Nature is rude and incom-
    prehensible at first,
Be not discouraged, keep on, there are divine things well envelop'd,
I swear to you there are divine things more beautiful than words can tell.

Allons! we must not stop here,
However sweet these laid-up stores, however convenient this dwelling we can-
    not remain here,
However shelter'd this port and however calm these waters we must not
    anchor here,
However welcome the hospitality that surrounds us we are permitted to
    receive it but a little while.

10

Allons! the inducements shall be greater,
We will sail pathless and wild seas,
We will go where winds blow, waves dash, and the Yankee clipper speeds by
    under full sail.

Allons! with power, liberty, the earth, the elements,
Health, defiance, gayety, self-esteem, curiosity;
Allons! from all formules!
From your formules, O bat-eyed and materialistic priests.

The stale cadaver blocks up the passage—the burial waits no longer.

Allons! yet take warning!
He traveling with me needs the best blood, thews, endurance,
None may come to the trial till he or she bring courage and health,
Come not here if you have already spent the best of yourself,

Only those may come who come in sweet and determin'd bodies,
No diseas'd person, no rum-drinker or venereal taint is permitted here.

(I and mine do not convince by arguments, similes, rhymes,
We convince by our presence.)

11
Listen! I will be honest with you,
I do not offer the old smooth prizes, but offer rough new prizes,
These are the days that must happen to you:
You shall not heap up what is call'd riches,
You shall scatter with lavish hand all that you earn or achieve,
You but arrive at the city to which you were destin'd, you hardly settle yourself
    to satisfaction before you are call'd by an irresistible call to depart,
You shall be treated to the ironical smiles and mockings of those who remain
    behind you,
What beckonings of love you receive you shall only answer with passionate
    kisses of parting,
You shall not allow the hold of those who spread their reach'd hands toward
    you.

12
Allons! after the great Companions, and to belong to them!
They too are on the road—they are the swift and majestic men—they are the
    greatest women,
Enjoyers of calms of seas and storms of seas,
Sailors of many a ship, walkers of many a mile of land,
Habitués of many distant countries, habitués of far-distant dwellings,

Trusters of men and women, observers of cities, solitary toilers,
Pausers and contemplators of tufts, blossoms, shells of the shore,
Dancers at wedding-dances, kissers of brides, tender helpers of children, bear-
    ers of children,
Soldiers of revolts, standers by gaping graves, lowerers-down of coffins,
Journeyers over consecutive seasons, over the years, the curious years each
    emerging from that which preceded it,

Journeyers as with companions, namely their own diverse phases,

Forth-steppers from the latent unrealized baby-days,

Journeyers gayly with their own youth, journeyers with their bearded and well-grain'd manhood,

Journeyers with their womanhood, ample, unsurpass'd, content,

Journeyers with their own sublime old age of manhood or womanhood,

Old age, calm, expanded, broad with the haughty breadth of the universe,

Old age, flowing free with the delicious near-by freedom of death.

13

Allons! to that which is endless as it was beginningless,

To undergo much, tramps of days, rests of nights,

To merge all in the travel they tend to, and the days and nights they tend to,

Again to merge them in the start of superior journeys,

To see nothing anywhere but what you may reach it and pass it,

To conceive no time, however distant, but what you may reach it and pass it,

To look up or down no road but it stretches and waits for you, however long but it stretches and waits for you,

To see no being, not God's or any, but you also go thither,

To see no possession but you may possess it, enjoying all without labor or purchase, abstracting the feast yet not abstracting one particle of it,

To take the best of the farmer's farm and the rich man's elegant villa, and the chaste blessings of the well-married couple, and the fruits of orchards and flowers of gardens,

To take to your use out of the compact cities as you pass through,

To carry buildings and streets with you afterward wherever you go,

To gather the minds of men out of their brains as you encounter them, to gather the love out of their hearts,

To take your lovers on the road with you, for all that you leave them behind you,

To know the universe itself as a road, as many roads, as roads for traveling souls.

All parts away for the progress of souls,

All religion, all solid things, arts, governments—all that was or is apparent upon this globe or any globe, falls into niches and corners before the procession of souls along the grand roads of the universe.

Of the progress of the souls of men and women along the grand roads of the
universe, all other progress is the needed emblem and sustenance.

Forever alive, forever forward,
Stately, solemn, sad, withdrawn, baffled, mad, turbulent, feeble, dissatisfied,
Desperate, proud, fond, sick, accepted by men, rejected by men,
They go! they go! I know that they go, but I know not where they go,
But I know that they go toward the best—toward something great.

Whoever you are, come forth! or man or woman come forth!
You must not stay sleeping and dallying there in the house, though you built
it, or though it has been built for you.

Out of the dark confinement! out from behind the screen!
It is useless to protest, I know all and expose it.

Behold through you as bad as the rest,
Through the laughter, dancing, dining, supping, of people,
Inside of dresses and ornaments, inside of those wash'd and trimm'd faces,
Behold a secret silent loathing and despair.

No husband, no wife, no friend, trusted to hear the confession,
Another self, a duplicate of every one, skulking and hiding it goes,
Formless and wordless through the streets of the cities, polite and bland in the
    parlors,
In the cars of railroads, in steamboats, in the public assembly,
Home to the houses of men and women, at the table, in the bedroom, every-
    where,
Smartly attired, countenance smiling, form upright, death under the breast-
    bones, hell under the skull-bones,
Under the broadcloth and gloves, under the ribbons and artificial flowers,
Keeping fair with the customs, speaking not a syllable of itself,
Speaking of any thing else but never of itself.

14

Allons! through struggles and wars!
The goal that was named cannot be countermanded.

Have the past struggles succeeded?
What has succeeded? yourself? your nation? Nature?
Now understand me well—it is provided in the essence of things that from
    any fruition of success, no matter what, shall come forth something to
    make a greater struggle necessary.

My call is the call of battle, I nourish active rebellion,
He going with me must go well arm'd,
He going with me goes often with spare diet, poverty, angry enemies, deser-
    tions.

15

Allons! the road is before us!
It is safe—I have tried it—my own feet have tried it well—be not detain'd!

Let the paper remain on the desk unwritten, and the book on the shelf
    unopen'd!
Let the tools remain in the workshop! let the money remain unearn'd!
Let the school stand! mind not the cry of the teacher!
Let the preacher preach in his pulpit! let the lawyer plead in the court, and the
    judge expound the law.

Camerado, I give you my hand!
I give you my love more precious than money,
I give you myself before preaching or law;
Will you give me yourself? will you come travel with me?
Shall we stick by each other as long as we live?

Kan'ami Kiyotsugu
SOTOBA KOMACHI

Translated by Sam Houston Brock

Persons
FIRST PRIEST
SECOND PRIEST
KOMACHI, as herself and as her former lover
CHORUS

BOTH PRIESTS: The mountains are not high on which we hide
The mountains are not high on which we hide
The lonely deepness of our hearts.
FIRST PRIEST: I am a priest from the Koya Hills
Coming down now to make my way to the city.
SECOND PRIEST: The Buddha that was is gone away.
The Buddha to be has not yet come to the world.
BOTH PRIESTS: At birth we woke to dream in this world between.
What then shall we say is real?
By chance we took the forms of men
From a thousand possibilities.
We stumbled on the treasure of the holy law
The seed of all salvation
And then with thoughtful hearts we put our bodies
In these thin and ink-black robes.
We knew of lives before this birth
We knew of lives before this birth
And knew we owed no love to those who to this life
Engendered us.
We recognized no parents.
No children cared for us.
We walked a thousand miles and the way seemed short.

In the fields we lay down
And slept the night in the hills
Which now became our proper dwelling place
Our proper home.
KOMACHI: "Like a root-cut reed
Should the tide entice
I would come
I would come I know but no wave asks
No stream invites this grief."
How sad that once I was proud
Long ago
Proud and graceful
Golden birds in my raven hair
When I walked like willows nodding, charming
As the breeze in spring.
The voice of the nightingale
The petals of the wood rose, wide stretched,
Holding dew
At the hour before their breathless fall:
I was lovelier than these.
Now
I am foul in the eyes of the humblest creatures
To whom my shame is shown.
Unwelcome months and days pile over me
The wreck of a hundred years
In the city to avoid the eyes of men
Lest they should say "Can it be she?"
In the evening
West with the moon I steal past the palace,
Past the towers
Where no guard will question in the mountains
In the shadows of the trees
None challenge so wretched a pilgrim as this
To Love's Tomb
The autumn hills
The River Katsura

Boats in the moonlight rowed by whom?

I cannot see. . . .

But rowed by whom!

Oh, too, too painful. . . .

Here on this withered stump of tree

Let me sit and collect my senses.

FIRST PRIEST: Come on. The sun is down. We must hurry on our way. But look! that old beggar woman sitting there on a sacred stupa. We should warn her to come away.

SECOND PRIEST: Yes, of course.

FIRST PRIEST: Excuse me, old lady, but don't you know that's a stupa there you're sitting on? the holy image of the Buddha's incarnation. You'd better come away and rest some other place.

KOMACHI: The holy image of the Buddha you say? But I saw no words or carvings on it. I took it for a tree stump only.

FIRST PRIEST: "Withered stumps

Are known as pine or cherry still

On the loneliest mountain."

KOMACHI: I, too, am a fallen tree.

But still the flowers of my heart

Might make some offering to the Buddha.

But this you call the Buddha's body. Why?

FIRST PRIEST: The stupa represents the body of Kongosatta Buddha, the Diamond Lord, when he assumed the temporary form of each of his manifestations.

KOMACHI: In what forms then is he manifested?

FIRST PRIEST: In Earth and Water and Wind and Fire and Space.

KOMACHI: The same five elements as man. What was the difference then?

FIRST PRIEST: The form was the same but not the power.

KOMACHI: And what is a stupa's power?

FIRST PRIEST: "He that has once looked upon a stupa shall for all eternity avoid the three worst catastrophes."

KOMACHI: "One sudden thought can strike illumination." Is that not just as good?

SECOND PRIEST: If you've had such an illumination, why are you lingering here in this world of illusion?

KOMACHI: Though my body lingers, my heart has left it long ago.

FIRST PRIEST: Unless you had no heart at all you wouldn't have failed to feel the presence of a stupa.

KOMACHI: It was because I felt it that I came perhaps.

SECOND PRIEST: In that case you shouldn't have spread yourself out on it without so much as a word of prayer.

KOMACHI: It was on the ground already. . . .

FIRST PRIEST: Just the same it was an act of discord.

KOMACHI: "Even from discord salvation springs."

SECOND PRIEST: From the evil of Daiba

KOMACHI: Or the love of Kannon.

FIRST PRIEST: From the folly of Handoku

KOMACHI: Or the wisdom of Monju.

FIRST PRIEST: What we call evil

KOMACHI: Is also good.

FIRST PRIEST: Illusion

KOMACHI: Is Salvation.

SECOND PRIEST: "Salvation

KOMACHI: Cannot be watered like trees."

FIRST PRIEST: "The brightest mirror

KOMACHI: Is not on the wall."

CHORUS: Nothing is separate.

Nothing persists.

Of Buddha and man there is no distinction,

At most a seeming difference planned

For the humble, ill-instructed men

He has vowed from the first to save.

"Even from discord salvation springs."

So said Komachi. And the priests:

"Surely this beggar is someone beyond us."

Then bending their heads to the ground

Three times did they do her homage

The difficult priests

The difficult priests

Who thought to correct her.

FIRST PRIEST: Who are you then? Give us your name; we will pray for your soul.

KOMACHI: For all my shame I will tell you. Pray for the wreck of Komachi, the daughter of Yoshizane of Ono, Lord of Dewa.

BOTH PRIESTS: How sad to think that you were she.

Exquisite Komachi
The brightest flower long ago
Her dark brows arched
Her face bright-powdered always
When cedar-scented halls could scarce contain
Her damask robes.

KOMACHI: I made verses in our speech
And in the speech of the foreign court.

CHORUS: When she passed the banquet cup
Reflected moonlight lay on her sleeve.
How was ever such loveliness lost?
When did she change?
Her hair a tangle of frosted grass
Where the black curls lay on her neck
And the color lost from the twin arched peaks
Of her brow.

KOMACHI: "Oh shameful in the dawning light
These silted seaweed locks that of a hundred years
Now lack but one."

CHORUS: What do you have in the bag at your waist?

KOMACHI: Death today or hunger tomorrow.
Only some beans I've put in my bag.

CHORUS: And in the bundle on your back?

KOMACHI: A soiled and dusty robe.

CHORUS: And in the basket on your arm?

KOMACHI: Sagittaries black and white.

CHORUS: Tattered coat

KOMACHI: Broken hat

CHORUS: Can scarcely hide her face.

KOMACHI: Think of the frost and the show and the rain.
I've not even sleeves enough to dry my tears.
But I wander begging things from men

That come and go along the road.
When begging fails
An awful madness seizes me
And my voice is no longer the same. . . .
   Hey! Give me something, you priests!
FIRST PRIEST: What do you want?
KOMACHI: To go to Komachi!
FIRST PRIEST: What are you saying? You *are* Komachi!
KOMACHI: No. Komachi was beautiful.
Many letters came, many messages
Thick as rain from a summer sky
But she made no answer, even once,
Even an empty word.
Age is her retribution now.
Oh, I love her!
I love her!
FIRST PRIEST: You love her! What spirit has possessed you to make you say
   such things?
KOMACHI: Many loved her
But among them all
It was Shosho who loved her deepest
Shii no Shosho, the Captain.
CHORUS: The wheel turns back.
I live again a cycle of unhappiness
Riding with the wheels
That came and went again each night.
The sun.
What time is it now?
Dusk.
The moon will be my friend on the road
And though the watchmen stand at the pass
They shall not bar my way.
KOMACHI (recostumed as her lover): My wide white skirts hitched up
CHORUS: My wide white skirts hitched up
My tall black hat pulled down
And my sleeves thrown over my head

Hidden from the eyes of men on the road
In the moonlight
In the darkness coming, coming
When the night rains fell
When the night winds blew the leaves like rain
When the snow lay deep
KOMACHI: And the melting drops fell
One by one from the rafters
CHORUS: I came and went, came and went
One night, two nights, three,
Ten (and this was the Harvest Night)
And did not see her.
Faithful as a cock that marks each dawn
I came and carved my mark upon the pillar.
I was to come a hundred nights,
I lacked but one. . . .
KOMACHI: Oh, dizziness . . . pain. . . .
CHORUS: He was grieved at the pain in his breast
When the last night came and he died
Shii no Shosho, the Captain.
KOMACHI: It was his unsatisfied love possessed me so
His anger that turned my wits.
In the face of this I will pray
For life in the worlds to come
The sands of goodness I will pile
Into a towering hill.
Before the golden, gentle Buddha I will lay
Poems as my flowers
Entering in the Way
Entering in the Way.

Frank O'Hara
A STEP AWAY FROM THEM

It's my lunch hour, so I go
for a walk among the hum-colored
cabs. First, down the sidewalk
where laborers feed their dirty
glistening torsos sandwiches
and Coca-Cola, with yellow helmets
on. They protect them from falling
bricks, I guess. Then onto the
avenue where skirts are flipping
above heels and blow up over
grates. The sun is hot, but the
cabs stir up the air. I look
at bargains in wristwatches. There
are cats playing in sawdust.
                         On
to Times Square, where the sign
blows smoke over my head, and higher
the waterfall pours lightly. A
Negro stands in a doorway with a
toothpick, languorously agitating.
A blonde chorus girl clicks; he
smiles and rubs his chin. Everything
suddenly honks: it is 12:40 of
a Thursday.
            Neon in daylight is a
great pleasure, as Edwin Denby would
write, as are light bulbs in daylight.
I stop for a cheeseburger at JULIET'S

CORNER. Giulietta Masina, wife of
Federico Fellini, *è bell' attrice.*
And chocolate malted. A lady in
foxes on such a day puts her poodle
in a cab.
        There are several Puerto
Ricans on the avenue today, which
makes it beautiful and warm. First
Bunny died, then John Latouche,
then Jackson Pollock. But is the
earth as full as life was full, of them?
And one has eaten and one walks,
past the magazines with nudes
and the posters for BULLFIGHT and
the Manhattan Storage Warehouse,
which they'll soon tear down. I
used to think they had the Armory
Show there.
        A glass of papaya juice
and back to work. My heart is in my
pocket, it is Poems by Pierre Reverdy.

Denise Levertov
STEPPING WESTWARD

What is green in me
darkens, muscadine.

If woman is inconstant,
good, I am faithful to

ebb and flow, I fall
in season and now

is a time of ripening.
If her part

is to be true,
a north star,

good, I hold steady
in the black sky

and vanish by day,
yet burn there

in blue or above
quilts of cloud.

There is no savor
more sweet, more salt

than to be glad to be
what, woman,

and who, myself,
I am, a shadow

that grows longer as the sun
moves, drawn out

on a thread of wonder.
If I bear burdens

they begin to be remembered
as gifts, goods, a basket

of bread that hurts
my shoulders but closes me

in fragrance. I can
eat as I go.

William Wordsworth
STEPPING WESTWARD

"What, you are stepping westward?"—"Yea."
—'Twould be a *wildish* destiny,
If we, who thus together roam
In a strange Land, and far from home,
Were in this place the guests of Chance:
Yet who would stop, or fear to advance,
Though home or shelter he had none,
With such a sky to lead him on?

The dewy ground was dark and cold;
Behind, all gloomy to behold;
And stepping westward seemed to be
A kind of *heavenly* destiny:
I liked the greeting; 'twas a sound
Of something without place or bound;
And seemed to give me spiritual right
To travel through that region bright.

The voice was soft, and she who spake
Was walking by her native lake:
The salutation had to me
The very sound of courtesy:
Its power was felt; and while my eye
Was fixed upon the glowing Sky,
The echo of the voice enwrought
A human sweetness with the thought
Of travelling through the world that lay
Before me in my endless way.

Virginia Woolf
STREET HAUNTING
A LONDON ADVENTURE

No one perhaps has ever felt passionately towards a lead pencil. But there are circumstances in which it can become supremely desirable to possess one; moments when we are set upon having an object, an excuse for walking half across London between tea and dinner. As the foxhunter hunts in order to preserve the breed of foxes, and the golfer plays in order that open spaces may be preserved from the builders, so when the desire comes upon us to go street rambling a pencil does for a pretext, and getting up we say: "Really I must buy a pencil," as if under cover of this excuse we could indulge safely in the greatest pleasure of town life in winter—rambling the streets of London.

The hour should be the evening and the season winter, for in winter the champagne brightness of the air and the sociability of the streets are grateful. We are not then taunted as in the summer by the longing for shade and solitude and sweet airs from the hayfields. The evening hour, too, gives us the irresponsibility which darkness and lamplight bestow. We are no longer quite ourselves. As we step out of the house on a fine evening between four and six, we shed the self our friends know us by and become part of that vast republican army of anonymous trampers, whose society is so agreeable after the solitude of one's own room, For there we sit surrounded by objects which perpetually express the oddity of our own temperaments and enforce the memories of our own experience. That bowl on the mantelpiece, for instance, was bought at Mantua on a windy day. We were leaving the shop when the sinister old woman plucked at our skirts and said she would find herself starving one of these days, but, "Take it!" she cried, and thrust the blue and white china bowl into our hands as if she never wanted to be reminded of her quixotic generosity. So, guiltily, but suspecting nevertheless how badly we had been fleeced, we carried it back to the little hotel where, in the middle of the night, the innkeeper quarrelled so violently with his wife that we all leant out into the courtyard to look, and saw the vines laced about among the pillars and the stars white in the sky. The moment was stabilized, stamped like a coin indelibly among a million that slipped by imperceptibly. There, too, was the melancholy Englishman, who rose among the coffee cups and the little iron tables and revealed the secrets of his soul—as travellers do. All this—Italy, the windy morning, the vines laced about the pillars, the Englishman and the secrets of his soul—rise up in a cloud from the china bowl on the mantelpiece. And there, as our eyes fall to the floor, is that brown stain on the carpet. Mr. Lloyd George made that. "The man's a devil!" said Mr. Cummings, putting the kettle down with which he was about to fill the teapot so that it burnt a brown ring on the carpet.

But when the door shuts on us, all that vanishes. The shell-like covering which our souls have excreted to house themselves, to make for themselves a shape distinct from others, is broken, and there is left of all these wrinkles and roughnesses a central oyster of perceptiveness, an enormous eye. How beautiful a street is in winter! It is at once revealed and obscured. Here vaguely one can trace symmetrical straight avenues of doors and windows; here under the lamps are floating islands of pale light through which pass quickly bright men and women, who, for all their poverty and shabbiness, wear a certain look of unreality, an air of triumph, as if they had given life the slip, so that life, deceived of her prey, blunders on without them. But, after all, we are only gliding smoothly on the surface. The eye is not a miner, not a diver, not a seeker after buried treasure. It floats us smoothly down a stream; resting, pausing, the brain sleeps perhaps as it looks.

How beautiful a London street is then, with its islands of light, and its long groves of darkness, and on one side of it perhaps some tree-sprinkled, grass-grown space where night is folding herself to sleep naturally and, as one passes the iron railing, one hears those little cracklings and stirrings of leaf and twig which seem to suppose the silence of fields all round them, an owl hooting, and far away the rattle of a train in the valley. But this is London, we are reminded; high among the bare trees are hung oblong frames of reddish yellow light—windows; there are points of brilliance burning steadily like low stars—lamps; this empty ground, which holds the country in it and its peace, is only a London square, set about by offices and houses where at this hour fierce lights burn over maps, over documents, over desks where clerks sit turning with wetted forefinger the files of endless correspondences; or more suffus-edly the firelight wavers and the lamplight falls upon the privacy of some drawing-room, its easy chairs, its papers, its china, its inlaid table, and the fig-ure of a woman, accurately measuring out the precise number of spoons of tea which— She looks at the door as if she heard a ring downstairs and somebody asking, is she in?

But here we must stop peremptorily. We are in danger of digging deeper than the eye approves; we are impeding our passage down the smooth stream by catching at some branch or root. At any moment, the sleeping army may stir itself and wake in us a thousand violins and trumpets in response; the army of human beings may rouse itself and assert all its oddities and sufferings and sordidities. Let us dally a little longer, be content still with surfaces only— the glossy brilliance of the motor omnibuses; the carnal splendour of the butchers' shops with their yellow flanks and purple steaks; the blue and red bunches of flowers burning so bravely through the plate glass of the florists' windows.

For the eye has this strange property: it rests only on beauty; like a butterfly it seeks colour and basks in warmth. On a winter's night like this, when nature has been at pains to polish and preen herself, it brings back the prettiest tro-phies, breaks off little lumps of emerald and coral as if the whole earth were made of precious stone. The thing it cannot do (one is speaking of the average unprofessional eye) is to compose these trophies in such a way as to bring out the more obscure angles and relationships. Hence after a prolonged diet of this simple, sugary fare, of beauty pure and uncomposed, we become conscious of satiety. We halt at the door of the boot shop and make some little excuse, which has nothing to do with the real reason, for folding up the bright para-phernalia of the streets and withdrawing to some duskier chamber of the being where we may ask, as we raise our left foot obediently upon the stand: "What, then, is it like to be a dwarf?"

She came in escorted by two women who, being of normal size, looked like benevolent giants beside her. Smiling at the shop girls, they seemed to be dis-claiming any lot in her deformity and assuring her of their protection. She wore the peevish yet apologetic expression usual on the faces of the deformed. She needed their kindness, yet she resented it. But when the shop girl had been summoned and the giantesses, smiling indulgently, had asked for shoes for "this lady" and the girl had pushed the little stand in front of her, the dwarf stuck her foot out with an impetuosity which seemed to claim all our attention. Look at that! Look at that! she seemed to demand of us all, as she thrust her foot out; for behold it was the shapely, perfectly proportioned foot of a well-grown woman. It was arched; it was aristocratic. Her whole manner changed as she looked at it resting on the stand. She looked soothed and satisfied. Her manner became full of self-confidence. She sent for shoe after shoe; she tried on pair after pair. She got up and pirouetted before a glass which reflected the foot only in yellow shoes, in fawn shoes, in shoes of lizard skin. She raised her little skirts and displayed her little legs. She was thinking that, after all, feet are the most important part of the whole person; women, she said to herself, have been loved for their feet alone. Seeing nothing but her feet, she imagined perhaps that the rest of her body was of a piece with those beautiful feet. She was shabbily dressed, but she was ready to lavish any money upon her shoes. And as this was the only occasion upon which she was not afraid of being looked at but positively craved attention, she was ready to use any device to prolong the choosing and fitting. Look at my feet, she seemed to be saying, as she took a step this way and then a step that way. The shop girl good-humouredly must have said something flattering, for suddenly her face lit up in ecstasy. But, after all, the giantesses, benevolent though they were, had their own affairs to see to; she must make up her mind; she must decide which to choose. At length, the pair was chosen and, as she walked out between her guardians, with the parcel swinging from her finger, the ecstasy faded, knowledge returned, the old peevishness, the old apology came back, and by the time she had reached the street again she had become a dwarf only.

But she had changed the mood; she had called into being an atmosphere which, as we followed her out into the street, seemed actually to create the humped, the twisted, the deformed. Two bearded men, brothers, apparently, stone-blind, supporting themselves by resting a hand on the head of a small boy between them, marched down the street. On they came with the unyielding yet tremulous tread of the blind, which seems to lend to their approach something of the terror and inevitability of the fate that has overtaken them. As they passed, holding straight on, the little convoy seemed to cleave asunder the passers-by with the momentum of its silence, its directness, its disaster. Indeed, the dwarf had started a hobbling grotesque dance to which everybody in the street now conformed: the stout lady tightly swathed in shiny sealskin; the feeble-minded boy sucking the silver knob of his stick; the old man squatted on a doorstep as if, suddenly overcome by the absurdity of the human spectacle, he had sat down to look at it—all joined in the hobble and tap of the dwarf's dance.

In what crevices and crannies, one might ask, did they lodge, this maimed company of the halt and the blind? Here, perhaps, in the top rooms of these narrow old houses between Holborn and Soho, where people have such queer names, and pursue so many curious trades, are gold beaters, accordion pleaters, cover buttons, or support life, with even great fantasticality, upon a traffic in cups without saucers, china umbrella handles, and highly-coloured pictures of martyred saints. There they lodge, and it seems as if the lady in the sealskin jacket must find life tolerable, passing the time of day with the accordion pleater, or the man who covers buttons; life which is so fantastic cannot be altogether tragic. They do not grudge us, we are musing, our prosperity; when, suddenly, turning the corner, we come upon a bearded Jew, wild, hunger-bitten, glaring out of his misery; or pass the humped body of an old woman flung abandoned on the step of a public building with a cloak over her like the hasty covering thrown over a dead horse or donkey. At such sights the nerves of the spine seem to stand erect; a sudden flare is brandished in our eyes; a question is asked which is never answered. Often enough these derelicts choose to lie not a stone's throw from theatres, within hearing of barrel organs, almost, as night draws on, within touch of the sequined cloaks and bright legs of diners and dancers. They lie close to those shop windows where commerce offers to a world of old women laid on doorsteps, of blind men, of hobbling dwarfs, sofas which are supported by the gilt necks of proud swans; tables inlaid with baskets of many coloured fruit; sideboards paved with green marble the better to support the weight of boars' heads; and carpets so softened with age that their carnations have almost vanished in a pale green sea.

Passing, glimpsing, everything seems accidentally but miraculously sprinkled with beauty, as if the tide of trade which deposits its burden so punctually and prosaically upon the shores of Oxford Street had this night cast up nothing but treasure. With no thought of buying, the eye is sportive and generous; it creates; it adorns; it enhances. Standing out in the street, one may build up all the chambers of an imaginary house and furnish them at one's will with sofa, table, carpet. That rug will do for the hall. That alabaster bowl shall stand on a carved table in the window. Our merrymaking shall be reflected in that thick round mirror. But, having built and furnished the house, one is happily under no obligation to possess it; one can dismantle it in the twinkling of an eye, and build and furnish another house with other chairs and other glasses. Or let us indulge ourselves at the antique jewellers, among the trays of rings and the hanging necklaces. Let us choose those pearls, for example, and then imagine how, if we put them on, life would be changed. It becomes instantly between two and three in the morning; the lamps are burning very white in the deserted streets of Mayfair. Only motor-cars are abroad at this hour, and one has a sense of emptiness, of airiness, of secluded gaiety. Wearing pearls, wearing silk, one steps out on to a balcony which overlooks the gardens of sleeping Mayfair. There are a few lights in the bedrooms of great peers returned from Court, of silk-stockinged footmen, of dowagers who have pressed the hands of statesmen. A cat creeps along the garden wall. Love-making is going on sibilantly, seductively in the darker places of the room behind thick green curtains. Strolling sedately as if he were promenading a terrace beneath which the shires and counties of England lie sun-bathed, the aged Prime Minister recounts to Lady So-and-So with the curls and the emeralds the true history of some great crisis in the affairs of the land. We seem to be riding on the top of the highest mast of the tallest ship; and yet at the same time we know that nothing of this sort matters; love is not proved thus, nor great achievements completed thus; so that we sport with the moment and preen our feathers in it lightly, as we stand on the balcony watching the moon-lit cat creep along Princess Mary's garden wall.

But what could be more absurd? It is, in fact, on the stroke of six; it is a winter's evening; we are walking to the Strand to buy a pencil. How, then, are we also on a balcony, wearing pearls in June? What could be more absurd? Yet it is nature's folly, not ours. When she set about her chief masterpiece, the making of man, she should have thought of one thing only. Instead, turning her head, looking over her shoulder, into each one of us she let creep instincts and desires which are utterly at variance with his being, so that we are streaked, variegated, all of a mixture; the colours have run. Is the true self this which stands on the pavement in January, or that which bends over the balcony in June? Am I here, or am I there? Or is the true self neither this nor that, neither here nor there, but something so varied and wandering that it is only when we give the rein to its wishes and let it take its way unimpeded that we are indeed ourselves? Circumstances compel unity; for convenience' sake a man must be a whole. The good citizen when he opens his door in the evening must be banker, golfer, husband, father; not a nomad wandering the desert, a mystic staring at the sky, a debauchee in the slums of San Francisco, a soldier heading a revolution, a pariah howling with scepticism and solitude. When he opens his door, he must run his fingers through his hair and put his umbrella in the stand like the rest.

But here, none too soon, are the second-hand bookshops. Here we find anchorage in these thwarting currents of being; here we balance ourselves after the splendours and miseries of the streets. The very sight of the bookseller's wife with her foot on the fender, sitting beside a good coal fire, screened from the door, is sobering and cheerful. She is never reading, or only the newspaper; her talk, when it leaves bookselling, which it does so gladly, is about hats; she likes a hat to be practical, she says, as well as pretty. O no, they don't live at the shop; they live in Brixton; she must have a bit of green to look at. In summer a jar of flowers grown in her own garden is stood on the top of some dusty pile to enliven the shop. Books are everywhere; and always the same sense of adventure fills us. Second-hand books are wild books, homeless books; they have come together in vast flocks of variegated feather, and have a charm which the domesticated volumes of the library lack. Besides, in this random miscellaneous company we may rub against some complete stranger who will, with luck, turn into the best friend we have in the world. There is always a hope, as we reach down some greyish-white book from an upper shelf, direct-ed by its air of shabbiness and desertion, of meeting here with a man who set out on horseback over a hundred years ago to explore the woollen market in the Midlands and Wales; an unknown traveller, who stayed at inns, drank his pint, noted pretty girls and serious customs, wrote it all down stiffly, laborious-ly for sheer love of it (the book was published at his own expense); was infi-nitely prosy, busy, and matter-of-fact, and so let flow in without his knowing it the very scent of hollyhocks and the hay together with such a portrait of him-self as gives him forever a seat in the warm corner of the mind's inglenook. One may buy him for eighteen pence now. He is marked three and sixpence, but the bookseller's wife, seeing how shabby the covers are and how long the book has stood there since it was bought at some sale of a gentleman's library in Suffolk, will let it go at that.

Thus, glancing round the bookshop, we make other such sudden capricious friendships with the unknown and the vanished whose only record is, for example, this little book of poems, so fairly printed, so finely engraved, too, with a portrait of the author. For he was a poet and drowned untimely, and his verse, mild as it is and formal and sententious, sends forth still a frail fluty sound like that of a piano organ played in some back street resignedly by an old Italian organ-grinder in a corduroy jacket. There are travellers, too, row upon row of them, still testifying, indomitable spinsters that they were, to the discomforts that they endured and the sunsets they admired in Greece when Queen Victoria was a girl. A tour in Cornwall with a visit to the tin mines was thought worthy of voluminous record. People went slowly up the Rhine and did portraits of each other in Indian ink, sitting reading on deck beside a coil of rope; they measured the pyramids; were lost to civilization for years; converted Negroes in pestilential swamps. This packing up and going off, exploring deserts and catching fevers, settling in India for a lifetime, penetrating even to China and then returning to lead a parochial life at Edmonton, tumbles and tosses upon the dusty floor like an uneasy sea, so restless the English are, with the waves at their very door. The waters of travel and adventure seem to break upon little islands of serious effort and lifelong industry stood in jagged column upon the floor. In these piles of puce-bound volumes with gilt monograms on the back, thoughtful clergymen expound the gospels; scholars are to be heard with their hammers and their chisels chipping clear the ancient texts of Euripides and Aeschylus. Thinking, annotating, expounding goes on at a prodigious rate all around us and over everything, like a punctual, everlasting tide, washes the ancient sea of fiction. Innumerable volumes tell how Arthur loved Laura and they were separated and they were unhappy and then they met and they were happy ever after, as was the way when Victoria ruled these islands.

The number of books in the world is infinite, and one is forced to glimpse and nod and move on after a moment of talk, a flash of understanding, as, in the street outside, one catches a word in passing and from a chance phrase fabricates a lifetime. It is about a woman called Kate that they are talking, how "I said to her quite straight last night . . . if you don't think I'm worth a penny stamp, I said . . ." But who Kate is, and to what crisis in their friendship that penny stamp refers, we shall never know; for Kate sinks under the warmth of their volubility; and here, at the street corner, another page of the volume of life is laid open by the sight of two men consulting under the lamp post. They are spelling out the latest wire from Newmarket in the stop press news. Do they think, then, that fortune will ever convert their rags into fur and broad-cloth, sling them with watch-chains, and plant diamond pins where there is now a ragged open shirt? But the main stream of walkers at this hour sweeps too fast to let us ask such questions. They are wrapt, in this short passage from work to home, in some narcotic dream, now that they are free from the desk, and have the fresh air on their cheeks. They put on those bright clothes which they must hang up and lock the key upon all the rest of the day, and are great cricketers, famous actresses, soldiers who have saved their country at the hour of need. Dreaming, gesticulating, often muttering a few words aloud, they sweep over the Strand and across Waterloo Bridge whence they will be slung in long rattling trains, to some prim little villa in Barnes or Surbiton where the sight of the clock in the hall and the smell of the supper in the basement puncture the dream.

But we are come to the Strand now, and as we hesitate on the curb, a little rod about the length of one's finger begins to lay its bar across the velocity and abundance of life. "Really I must—really I must"—that is it. Without investigating the demand, the mind cringes to the accustomed tyrant. One must, one always must, do something or other; it is not allowed one simply to enjoy oneself. Was it not for this reason that, some time ago, we fabricated the excuse, and invented the necessity of buying something? But what was it? Ah, we remember, it was a pencil. Let us go then and buy this pencil. But just as we are turning to obey the command, another self disputes the right of the tyrant to insist. The usual conflict comes about. Spread out behind the rod of duty we see the whole breadth of the river Thames—wide, mournful, peaceful. And we see it through the eyes of somebody who is leaning over the Embankment on a summer evening, without a care in the world. Let us put off buying the pencil; let us go in search of this person—and soon it becomes apparent that this person is ourselves. For if we could stand there where we stood six months ago, should we not be again as we were then—calm, aloof, content? Let us try then. But the river is rougher and greyer than we remembered. The tide is running out to sea. It brings down with it a tug and two barges, whose load of straw is tightly bound down beneath tarpaulin covers. There is, too, close by us, a couple leaning over the balustrade with the curious lack of self-consciousness lovers have, as if the importance of the affair they are engaged on claims without question the indulgence of the human race. The sights we see and the sounds we hear now have none of the quality of the past; nor have we any share in the serenity of the person who, six months ago, stood precisely where we stand now. His is the happiness of death; ours the insecurity of life. He has no future; the future is even now invading our peace. It is only when we look at the past and take from it the element of uncertainty that we can enjoy perfect peace. As it is, we must turn, we must cross the Strand again, we must find a shop where, even at this hour, they will be ready to sell us a pencil.

It is always an adventure to enter a new room; for the lives and characters of its owners have distilled their atmosphere into it, and directly we enter it we breast some new wave of emotion. Here, without a doubt, in the stationer's shop people had been quarrelling. Their anger shot through the air. They both stopped; the old woman—they were husband and wife evidently—retired to a back room; the old man whose rounded forehead and globular eyes would have looked well on the frontispiece of some Elizabethan folio, stayed to serve us. "A pencil, a pencil," he repeated, "certainly, certainly." He spoke with the distraction yet effusiveness of one whose emotions have been roused and checked in full flood. He began opening box after box and shutting them again. He said that it was very difficult to find things when they kept so many different articles. He launched into a story about some legal gentleman who had got into deep waters owing to the conduct of his wife. He had known him for years; he had been connected with the Temple for half a century, he said, as if he wished his wife in the back room to overhear him. He upset a box of rubber bands. At last, exasperated by his incompetence, he pushed the swing door open and called out roughly: "Where d'you keep the pencils?" as if his wife had hidden them. The old lady came in. Looking at nobody, she put her hand with a fine air of righteous severity upon the right box. There were pencils. How then could he do without her? Was she not indispensable to him? In order to keep them there, standing side by side in forced neutrality, one had to be particular in one's choice of pencils; this was too soft, that too hard. They stood silently looking on. The longer they stood there, the calmer they grew; their heat was going down, their anger disappearing. Now, without a word said on either side, the quarrel was made up. The old man, who would not have disgraced Ben Jonson's title-page, reached the box back to its proper place, bowed profoundly his good-night to us, and they disappeared. She would get out her sewing; he would read his newspaper; the canary would scatter them impartially with seed. The quarrel was over.

In these minutes in which a ghost has been sought for, a quarrel composed, and a pencil bought, the streets had become completely empty. Life had withdrawn to the top floor, and lamps were lit. The pavement was dry and hard; the road was of hammered silver. Walking home through the desolation one could tell oneself the story of the dwarf, of the blind men, of the party in the Mayfair mansion, of the quarrel in the stationer's shop. Into each of these lives one could penetrate a little way, far enough to give oneself the illusion that one is not tethered to a single mind, but can put on briefly for a few minutes the bodies and minds of others. One could become a washerwoman, a publican, a street singer. And what greater delight and wonder can there be than to leave the straight lines of personality and deviate into those footpaths that lead beneath brambles and thick tree trunks into the heart of the forest where live those wild beasts, our fellow men?

That is true: to escape is the greatest of pleasures; street haunting in winter the greatest of adventures. Still as we approach our own doorstep again, it is comforting to feel the old possessions, the old prejudices, fold us round; and the self, which has been blown about at so many street corners, which has battered like a moth at the flame of so many inaccessible lanterns, sheltered and enclosed. Here again is the usual door; here the chair turned as we left it and the china bowl and the brown ring on the carpet. And here—let us examine it tenderly, let us touch it with reverence—is the only spoil we have retrieved from all the treasures of the city, a lead pencil.

Franz Kafka
THE SUDDEN WALK

Translated by Willa and Edwin Muir

When it looks as if you had made up your mind finally to stay at home for the evening, when you have put on your house jacket and sat down after supper with a light on the table to the piece of work or the game that usually precedes your going to bed, when the weather outside is unpleasant so that staying indoors seems natural, and when you have already been sitting quietly at the table for so long that your departure must occasion surprise to everyone, when, besides, the stairs are in darkness and the front door locked, and in spite of all that you have started up in a sudden fit of restlessness, changed your jacket, abruptly dressed yourself for the street, explained that you must go out and with a few curt words of leave-taking actually gone out, banging the flat door more or less hastily according to the degree of displeasure you think you have left behind you, and when you find yourself once more in the street with limbs swinging extra freely in answer to the unexpected liberty you have procured for them, when as a result of this decisive action you feel concentrated within yourself all the potentialities of decisive action, when you recognize with more than usual significance that your strength is greater than your need to accomplish effortlessly the swiftest of changes and to cope with it, when in this frame of mind you go striding down the long streets—then for that evening you have completely got away from your family, which fades into insubstantiality, while you yourself, a firm, boldly drawn black figure, slapping yourself on the thigh, grow to your true stature.

All this is still heightened if at such a late hour in the evening you look up a friend to see how he is getting on.

Charles Reznikoff
SUNDAY WALKS IN THE SUBURBS

On stones mossed with hot dust, no shade but the thin, useless shadows of
    roadside grasses;
into the wood's gloom, staring back at the blue flowers on stalks thin as
    threads.

The green slime—a thicket of young trees standing in brown water;
with knobs like muscles, a naked tree stretches up,
dead; and a dead duck, head sunk in the water as if diving.

The tide is out. Only a pool is left on the creek's stinking mud.
Someone has thrown a washboiler away.
On the bank a heap of cans;
rats, covered with rust, creep in and out.
The white edges of the clouds like veining in a stone.

Allen Ginsberg
A SUPERMARKET IN CALIFORNIA

What thoughts I have of you tonight, Walt Whitman, for I walked down the sidestreets under the trees with a headache self-conscious looking at the full moon.

In my hungry fatigue, and shopping for images, I went into the neon fruit supermarket, dreaming of your enumerations!

What peaches and what penumbras! Whole families shopping at night! Aisles full of husbands! Wives in the avocados, babies in the tomatoes! —and you, García Lorca, what were you doing down by the watermelons?

I saw you, Walt Whitman, childless, lonely old grubber, poking among the meats in the refrigerator and eyeing the grocery boys.

I heard you asking questions of each: Who killed the pork chops? What price bananas? Are you my Angel?

I wandered in and out of the brilliant stacks of cans following you, and followed in my imagination by the store detective.

We strode down the open corridors together in our solitary fancy tasting artichokes, possessing every frozen delicacy, and never passing the cashier.

Where are we going, Walt Whitman? The doors close in an hour. Which way does your beard point tonight?

(I touch your book and dream of our odyssey in the supermarket and feel absurd.)

Will we walk all night through solitary streets? The trees add shade to shade, lights out in the houses, we'll both be lonely.

Will we stroll dreaming of the lost America of love past blue automobiles in driveways, home to our silent cottage?

Ah, dear father, graybeard, lonely old courage-teacher, what America did you have when Charon quit poling his ferry and you got out on a smoking bank and stood watching the boat disappear on the black waters of Lethe?

Marcel Proust
FROM SWANN'S WAY

That sense of the complexity of the Bois de Boulogne which made it an artificial place and, in the zoological or mythological sense of the word, a Garden, I captured again, this year, as I crossed it on my way to Trianon, on one of those mornings, early in November, when in Paris, if we stay indoors, being so near and yet prevented from witnessing the transformation scene of autumn, which is drawing so rapidly to a close without our assistance, we feel a regret for the fallen leaves that becomes a fever, and may even keep us awake at night. Into my closed room they had been drifting already for a month, summoned there by my desire to see them, slipping between my thoughts and the object, whatever it might be, upon which I was trying to concentrate them, whirling in front of me like those brown spots that sometimes, whatever we may be looking at, will seem to be dancing or swimming before our eyes. And on that morning, not hearing the splash of the rain as on the previous days, seeing the smile of fine weather at the corners of my drawn curtains, as from the corners of closed lips may escape the secret of their happiness, I had felt that I could actually see those yellow leaves, with the light shining through them, in their supreme beauty; and being no more able to restrain myself from going to look at the trees than, in my childhood's days, when the wind howled in the chimney, I had been able to resist the longing to visit the sea, I had risen and left the house to go to Trianon, passing through the Bois de Boulogne. It was the hour and the season in which the Bois seems, perhaps, most multiform, not only because it is then most divided, but because it is divided in a different way. Even in the unwooded parts, where the horizon is large, here and there against the background of a dark and distant mass of trees, now leafless or still keeping their summer foliage unchanged, a double row of orange-red chestnuts seemed, as in a picture just begun, to be the only thing painted, so far, by an artist who had not yet laid any colour on the rest, and to be offering their cloister, in full daylight, for the casual exercise of the human figures that would be added to the picture later on.

Farther off, at a place where the trees were still all green, one alone, small, stunted, lopped, but stubborn in its resistance, was tossing in the breeze an ugly mane of red. Elsewhere, again, might be seen the first awakening of this Maytime of the leaves, and those of an ampelopsis, a smiling miracle, like a red hawthorn flowering in winter, had that very morning all 'come out,' so to speak, in blossom. And the Bois had the temporary, unfinished, artificial look of a nursery garden or a park in which, either for some botanic purpose or hi preparation for a festival, there have been embedded among the trees of commoner growth, which have not yet been uprooted and transplanted elsewhere, a few rare specimens, with fantastic foliage, which seem to be clearing all round themselves an empty space, making room, giving air, diffusing light. Thus it was the time of year at which the Bois de Boulogne displays more separate characteristics, assembles more distinct elements in a composite whole than at any other. It was also the time of day. In places where the trees still kept their leaves, they seemed to have undergone an alteration of their substance from the point at which they were touched by the sun's light, still, at this hour in the morning, almost horizontal, as it would be again, a few hours later, at the moment when, just as dusk began, it would flame up like a lamp, project afar over the leaves a warm and artificial glow, and set ablaze the few topmost boughs of a tree that would itself remain unchanged, a sombre incombustible candelabrum beneath its flaming crest. At one spot the light grew solid as a brick wall, and like a piece of yellow Persian masonry, patterned in blue, daubed coarsely upon the sky the leaves of the chestnuts; at another, it cut them off from the sky towards which they stretched out their curling, golden fingers. Half-way up the trunk of a tree draped with wild vine, the light had grafted and brought to blossom, too dazzling to be clearly distinguished, an enormous posy, of red flowers apparently, perhaps of a new variety of carnation. The different parts of the Bois, so easily confounded in summer in the density and monotony of their universal green, were now clearly divided. A patch of brightness indicated the approach to almost every one of them, or else a splendid mass of foliage stood out before it like an oriflamme. I could make out, as on a coloured map, Armenonville, the Pré Catalan, Madrid, the Race Course and the shore of the lake. Here and there would appear some meaningless erection, a sham grotto, a mill, for which the trees made room by drawing away from it, or which was borne upon the soft green platform of a grassy lawn. I could feel that the Bois was not really a wood, that it existed for a purpose alien to the life of its trees; my sense of exaltation was due not only to admiration of the autumn tints but to a bodily desire. Ample source of a joy which the heart feels at first without being conscious of its cause, without understanding that it results from no external impulse! Thus I gazed at the trees with an unsatisfied longing which went beyond them and, without my knowledge, directed itself towards that masterpiece of beautiful strolling women which the trees enframed for a few hours every day. I walked towards the Allée des Acacias. I passed through forest groves in which the morning light, breaking them into new sections, lopped and trimmed the trees, united different trunks in marriage, made nosegays of their branches. It would skilfully draw towards it a pair of trees; making deft use of the sharp chisel of light and shade, it would cut away from each of them half of its trunk and branches, and, weaving together the two halves that remained, would make of them either a single pillar of shade, defined by the surrounding light, or a single luminous phantom whose artificial, quivering contour was encompassed in a network of inky shadows. When a ray of sunshine gilded the highest branches, they seemed, soaked and still dripping with a sparkling moisture, to have emerged alone from the liquid, emerald-green atmosphere in which the whole grove was plunged as though beneath the sea. For the trees continued to live by their own vitality, and when they had no longer any leaves, that vitality gleamed more brightly still from the nap of green velvet that carpeted their trunks, or in the white enamel of the globes of mistletoe that were scattered all the way up to the topmost branches of the poplars, rounded as are the sun and moon in Michelangelo's 'Creation.' But, forced for so many years now, by a sort of grafting process, to share the life of feminine humanity, they called to my mind the figure of the dryad, the fair worldling, swiftly walking, brightly coloured, whom they sheltered with their branches as she passed beneath them, and obliged to acknowledge, as they themselves acknowledged, the power of the season; they recalled to me the happy days when I was young and had faith, when I would hasten eagerly to the spots where masterpieces of female elegance would be incarnate for a few moments beneath the unconscious, accommodating boughs. But the beauty for which the firs and acacias of the Bois de Boulogne made me long, more disquieting in that respect than the chestnuts and lilacs of Trianon which I was going to see, was not fixed somewhere outside myself in the relics of an historical period, in works of art, in a little temple of love at whose door was piled an oblation of autumn leaves ribbed with gold. I reached the shore of the lake; I walked on as far as the pigeon-shooting ground. The idea of perfection which I had within me I had bestowed, in that other time, upon the height of a victoria, upon the raking thinness of those horses, frenzied and light as wasps upon the wing, with bloodshot eyes like the cruel steeds of Diomed, which now, smitten by a desire to see again what I had once loved, as ardent as the desire that had driven me, many years before, along the same paths, I wished to see renewed before my eyes at the moment when Mme. Swann's enormous coachman, supervised by a groom no bigger than his fist, and as infantile as Saint George in the picture, endeavoured to curb the ardour of, the flying, steel-tipped pinions with which they thundered along the ground. Alas! there was nothing now but motor-cars driven each by a moustached mechanic, with a tall footman towering by his side. I wished to hold before my bodily eyes, that I might know whether they were indeed as charming as they appeared to the eyes of memory, little hats, so low-crowned as to seem no more than garlands about the brows of women. All the hats now were immense, covered with fruits and flowers and all manner of birds. In place of the lovely gowns in which Mme. Swann walked like a Queen, appeared Greco-Saxon tunics, with Tanagra folds, or sometimes, in the Directoire style, 'Liberty chiffons' sprinkled with flowers like sheets of wallpaper. On the heads of the gentlemen who might have been eligible to stroll with Mme. Swann in the Allée de la Reine Marguerite, I found not the grey 'tile' hats of old, nor any other kind. They walked the Bois bare-headed. And seeing all these new elements of the spectacle, I had no longer the faith which, applied to them, would have given them consistency, unity, life; they passed in a scattered sequence before me, at random, without reality, containing in themselves no beauty that my eyes might have endeavoured, as in the old days, to extract from them and to compose in a picture. They were just women, in whose elegance I had no belief, and whose clothes seemed to me unimportant. But when a belief vanishes, there survives it—more and more ardently, so as to cloak the absence of the power, now lost to us, of imparting reality to new phenomena—an idolatrous attachment to the old things which our belief in them did once animate, as if it was in that belief and not in ourselves that the divine spark resided, and as if our present incredulity had a contingent cause—

the death of the gods.

"Oh, horrible!" I exclaimed to myself: "Does anyone really imagine that these motor-cars are as smart as the old carriage-and-pair? I dare say, I am too old now—but I was not intended for a world in which women shackle themselves in garments that are not even made of cloth. To what purpose shall I walk among these trees if there is nothing left now of the assembly that used to meet beneath the delicate tracery of reddening leaves, if vulgarity and fatuity have supplanted the exquisite thing that once their branches framed? Oh, horrible! My consolation is to think of the women whom I have known, in the past, now that there is no standard left of elegance. But how can the people who watch these dreadful creatures hobble by, beneath hats on which have been heaped the spoils of aviary or garden-bed,—how can they imagine the charm that there was in the sight of Mme. Swann, crowned with a close-fitting lilac bonnet, or with a tiny hat from which rose stiffly above her head a single iris?" Could I ever have made them understand the emotion that I used to feel on winter mornings, when I met Mme. Swann on foot, in an otter-skin coat, with a woollen cap from which stuck out two blade-like partridge-feathers, but enveloped also in the deliberate, artificial warmth of her own house, which was suggested by nothing more than the bunch of violets crushed into her bosom, whose flowering, vivid and blue against the grey sky, the freezing air, the naked boughs, had the same charming effect of using the season and the weather merely as a setting, and of living actually in a human atmosphere, in the atmosphere of this woman, as had in the vases and beaupots of her drawing-room, beside the blazing fire, in front of the silk-covered sofa, the flowers that looked out through closed windows at the falling snow? But it would not have sufficed me that the costumes alone should still have been the same as in those distant years. Because of the solidarity that binds together the different parts of a general impression, parts that our memory keeps in a balanced whole, of which we are not permitted to subtract or to decline any fraction, I should have liked to be able to pass the rest of the day with one of those women, over a cup of tea, in a little house with dark-painted walls (as Mme. Swann's were still in the year after that in which the first part of this story ends) against which would glow the orange flame, the red combustion, the pink and white flickering of her chrysanthemums in the twilight of a November evening, in moments similar to those in which (as we shall see) I had not managed to discover the pleasures for which I longed. But now, albeit they had led to nothing, those moments struck me as having been charming enough in themselves. I sought to find them again as I remembered them. Alas! there was nothing now but flats decorated in the Louis XVI style, all white paint, with hortensias in blue enamel. Moreover, people did not return to Paris, now, until much later. Mme. Swann would have written to me, from a country house, that she would not be in town before February, had I asked her to reconstruct for me the elements of that memory which I felt to belong to a distant era, to a date in time towards which it was forbidden me to ascend again the fatal slope, the elements of that longing which had become, itself, as inaccessible as the pleasure that it had once vainly pursued. And I should have required also that they be the same women, those whose costume interested me because, at a time when I still had faith, my imagination had individualised them and had provided each of them with a legend. Alas! in the acacia-avenue—the myrtle-alley—I did see some of them again, grown old, no more now than grim spectres of what once they had been, wandering to and fro, in desperate search of heaven knew what, through the Virgilian groves. They had long fled, and still I stood vainly questioning the deserted paths. The sun's face was hidden. Nature began again to reign over the Bois, from which had vanished all trace of the idea that it was the Elysian Garden of Woman; above the gimcrack windmill the real sky was grey; the wind wrinkled the surface of the Grand Lac in little wavelets, like a real lake; large birds passed swiftly over the Bois, as over a real wood, and with shrill cries perched, one after another, on the great oaks which, beneath their Druidical crown, and with Dodonaic majesty, seemed to proclaim the unpeopled vacancy of this estranged forest, and helped me to understand how paradoxical it is to seek in reality for the pictures that are stored in one's memory, which must inevitably lose the charm that comes to them from memory itself and from their not being apprehended by the senses. The reality that I had known no longer existed. It sufficed that Mme. Swann did not appear, in the same attire and at the same moment, for the whole avenue to be altered. The places that we have known belong now only to the little world of space on which we map them for our own convenience. None of them was ever more than a thin slice, held between the contiguous impressions that composed our life at that time; remembrance of a particular form is but regret for a particular moment; and houses, roads, avenues are as fugitive, alas, as the years.

Hugh Walpole
THE TARN

I

As Foster moved unconsciously across the room, bent towards the bookcase, and stood leaning forward a little, choosing now one book, now another with his eye, his host, seeing the muscles of the back of his thin, scraggy neck stand out above his low flannel collar, thought of the ease with which he could squeeze that throat and the pleasure, the triumphant, lustful pleasure, that such an action would give him.

The low white-walled, white-ceilinged room was flooded with the mellow, kindly Lakeland sun. October is a wonderful month in the English Lakes, golden, rich, and perfumed, slow suns moving through apricot-tinted skies to ruby evening glories; the shadows lie then thick about that beautiful country, in dark purple patches, in long web-like patterns of silver gauze, in thick splotches of amber and grey. The clouds pass in galleons across the mountains, now veiling, now revealing, now descending with ghost-like armies to the very breast of the plains, suddenly rising to the softest of blue skies and lying thin in lazy languorous colour.

Fenwick's cottage looked across to Low Fells; on his right, seen through side windows, sprawled the hills above Ullswater.

Fenwick looked at Foster's back and felt suddenly sick, so that he sat down, veiling his eyes for a moment with his hand. Foster had come up there, come all the way from London, to explain, to want to put things right. For how many years had he known Foster? Why, for twenty at least, and during all those years Foster had been for ever determined to put things right with everybody. He could not bear to be disliked; he hated that anyone should think ill of him; he wanted everyone to be his friend. That was one reason, perhaps, why Foster had got on so well, had prospered so in his career; one reason, too, why Fenwick had not.

For Fenwick was the opposite of Foster in this. He did not want friends; he certainly did not care that people should like him—that is, people for whom, for one reason or another, he had contempt—and he had contempt for quite a number of people.

Fenwick looked at that long, thin, bending back and felt his knees tremble. Soon Foster would turn round and that high reedy voice would pipe out something about the books. "What jolly books you have, Fenwick!" How many, many times in the long watches of the night when Fenwick could not sleep had he heard that pipe sounding close there—yes, in the very shadows of his bed! And how many times had Fenwick replied to it: "I hate you! You are the cause of my failure in life! You have been in my way always. Always, always, always! Patronising and pretending, and in truth showing others what a poor thing you thought me, how great a failure, how conceited a fool! I know. You can hide nothing from me! I can hear you!"

For twenty years now Foster had been persistently in Fenwick's way. There had been that affair, so long ago now, when Robins had wanted a sub-editor for his wonderful review, the *Parthenon,* and Fenwick had gone to see him and they had had a splendid talk. How magnificently Fenwick had talked that day, with what enthusiasm he had shown Robins (who was blinded by his own conceit, anyway) the kind of paper the *Parthenon* might be; how Robins had caught his own enthusiasm, how he had pushed his fat body about the room, crying, "Yes, yes, Fenwick—that's fine! That's fine indeed!"—and then how, after all, Foster had got that job.

The paper had only lived for a year or so, it is true, but the connection with it had brought Foster into prominence just as it might have brought Fenwick!

Then five years later there was Fenwick's novel, *The Bitter Aloe*—the novel upon which he had spent three years of blood-and-tears endeavour—and then, in the very same week of publication, Foster brings out *The Circus,* the novel that made his name, although, Heaven knows, the thing was poor sentimental trash. You may say that one novel cannot kill another—but can it not? Had not *The Circus* appeared would not that group of London know-alls— that conceited, limited, ignorant, self-satisfied crowd, who nevertheless can do, by their talk, so much to affect a book's good or evil fortunes—have talked about *The Bitter Aloe,* and so forced it into prominence? As it was, the book was still-born, and *The Circus* went on its prancing, triumphant way.

After that there had been many occasions—some small, some big—and always in one way or another that thin, scraggy body of Foster's was interfering with Fenwick's happiness.

The thing had become, of course, an obsession with Fenwick. Hiding up there in the heart of the Lakes, with no friends, almost no company, and very little money, he was given too much to brooding over his failure. He *was* a failure, and it was not his own fault. How could it be his own fault with his talents and his brilliance? It was the fault of modern life and its lack of culture, the fault of the stupid material mess that made up the intelligence of human beings—and the fault of Foster.

Always Fenwick hoped that Foster would keep away from him. He did not know what he would not do did he see the man. And then one day to his amazement he received a telegram: "Passing through this way. May I stop with you Monday and Tuesday? Giles Foster."

Fenwick could scarcely believe his eyes, and then—from curiosity, from cynical contempt, from some deeper, more mysterious motive that he dared not analyse—he had telegraphed "Come." And here the man was. And he had come—would you believe it?—to "put things right." He had heard from Hamlin Eddis that "Fenwick was hurt with him, had some kind of a grievance."

"I didn't like to feel that, old man, and so I thought I'd just stop by and have it out with you, see what the matter was, and put it right."

Last night after supper Foster had tried to put it right. Eagerly, his eyes like a good dog's who is asking for a bone that he knows that he thoroughly deserves, he had held out his hand and asked Fenwick to "say what was up."

Fenwick simply had said that nothing was up; Hamlin Eddis was a damned fool.

"Oh, I'm glad to hear that!" Foster had cried, springing out of his chair and putting his hand on Fenwick's shoulder. "I'm glad of that, old man. I couldn't bear for us not to be friends. We've been friends so long."

Lord, how Fenwick hated him at that moment!

II

"What a jolly lot of books you have!" Foster turned round and looked at Fenwick with eager, gratified eyes. "Every book here is interesting! I like your arrangement of them too, and those open bookshelves—it always seems to me a shame to shut up books behind glass!"

Foster came forward and sat down quite close to his host. He even reached forward and laid his hand on his host's knee. "Look here! I'm mentioning it for the last time—positively! But I do want to make quite certain. There *is* nothing wrong between us, is there, old man? I know you assured me last night, but I just want—"

Fenwick looked at him and, surveying him, felt suddenly an exquisite pleasure of hatred. He liked the touch of the man's hand on his knee; he himself bent forward a little and, thinking how agreeable it would be to push Foster's eyes in, deep, deep into his head, crunching them, smashing them to purple, leaving the empty, staring, bloody sockets, said:

Why, no. Of course not. I told you last night. What could there be?

The hand gripped the knee a little more tightly.

"I *am* so glad! That's splendid! Splendid! I hope you won't think me ridiculous, but I've always had an affection for you ever since I can remember. I've always wanted to know you better. I've admired your talents so greatly. That novel of yours—the—the—the one about the Aloe—"

"The Bitter Aloe?"

"Ah, yes, that was it. That was a splendid book. Pessimistic, of course, but still fine. It ought to have done better. I remember thinking so at the time."

"Yes, it ought to have done better."

"Your time will come, though. What I say is that good work always tells in the end."

"Yes, my time will come."

The thin, piping voice went on:

"Now, I've had more success than I deserved. Oh, yes, I have. You can't deny it. I'm not being falsely modest. I mean it. I've got some talent, of course, but not so much as people say. And you! Why, you've got so much *more* than they acknowledge. You have, old man. You have indeed. Only—I do hope you'll forgive my saying this—perhaps you haven't advanced quite as you might have done. Living up here, shut away here, closed in by all these mountains, in this wet climate—always raining—why, you're out of things! You don't see people, don't talk and discover what's really going on. Why, look at me!"

Fenwick turned round and looked at him.

"Now, I have half the year in London, where one gets the best of every-thing, best talk, best music, best plays, and then I'm three months abroad, Italy or Greece or somewhere, and then three months in the country. Now that's an ideal arrangement. You have everything that way."

"Italy or Greece or somewhere!"

Something turned in Fenwick's breast, grinding, grinding, grinding. How he had longed, oh, how passionately, for just one week in Greece, two days in Sicily! Sometimes he had thought that he might run to it, but when it had come to the actual counting of the pennies—and now this fool, this fathead, this self-satisfied, conceited, patronising—

He got up, looking out at the golden sun.

"What do you say to a walk?" he suggested. "The sun will last for a good hour yet."

III

As soon as the words were out of his lips he felt as though someone else had said them for him. He even turned half-round to see whether anyone else were there. Ever since Foster's arrival on the evening before he had been conscious of this sensation. A walk? Why should he take Foster for a walk, show him his beloved country, point out those curves and lines and hollows, the long silver shield of Ullswater, the cloudy purple hills hunched like blankets about the knees of some recumbent giant? Why? It was as though he had turned round to someone behind him and had said, "You have some further design in this."

They started out. The road sank abruptly to the lake, then the path ran between trees at the water's edge. Across the lake, tones of bright yellow light, crocus-hued, rode upon the blue. The hills were dark.

The very way that Foster walked bespoke the man. He was always a little ahead of you, pushing his long, thin body along with little eager jerks as though did he not hurry he would miss something that would be immensely to his advantage. He talked, throwing words over his shoulder to Fenwick as you throw crumbs of bread to a robin.

"Of course I was pleased. Who would not be? After all it's a new prize. They've only been awarding it for a year or two, but it's gratifying—really gratifying—to secure it. When I opened the envelope and found the cheque there—well, you could have knocked me down with a feather. You could, indeed. Of course, a hundred pounds isn't much. But it's the honour—"

Whither were they going? Their destiny was as certain as though they had no free-will. Free-will? There is no free-will. All is Fate. Fenwick suddenly laughed aloud.

Foster stopped.

"Why, what is it?"

"What's what?"

"You laughed."

"Something amused me."

Foster slipped his arm through Fenwick's.

"It *is* jolly to be walking alone together like this, arm-in-arm, friends. I'm a sentimental man, I won't deny it. What I say is that life is short and one must love one's fellow-beings or where is one? You live too much alone, old man." He squeezed Fenwick's arm. "That's the truth of it."

It was torture, exquisite, heavenly torture. It was wonderful to feel that thin, bony arm pressing against his. Almost you could hear the beating of that other heart. Wonderful to feel that arm and the temptation to take it in your two hands and to bend it and twist it and then to hear the bones crack . . . crack . . . crack. . . . Wonderful to feel that temptation rise through one's body like boiling water and yet not to yield to it. For a moment Fenwick's hand touched Foster's. Then he drew himself apart.

"We're at the village. This is the hotel where they all come in the summer. We turn off at the right here. I'll show you my tarn."

IV

"Your tarn?" asked Foster. "Forgive my ignorance, but what *is* a tarn exactly?"

"A tarn is a miniature lake, a pool of water lying in the lap of the hill. Very quiet, lovely, silent. Some of them are immensely deep."

"I should like to see that."

"It is some little distance—up a rough road. Do you mind?"

"Not a bit. I have long legs."

"Some of them are immensely deep—unfathomable—nobody touched the bottom—but quiet, like glass, with shadows only—"

"Do you know, Fenwick, but I have always been afraid of water—I've never learnt to swim. I'm afraid to go out of my depth. Isn't that ridiculous? But it is all because at my private school, years ago, when I was a small boy, some big fellows took me and held me with my head under the water and nearly drowned me. They did indeed. They went further than they meant to. I can see their faces."

Fenwick considered this. The picture leapt to his mind. He could see the boys—large, strong fellows, probably—and this little skinny thing like a frog, their thick hands about his throat, his legs like grey sticks kicking out of the water, their laughter, their sudden sense that something was wrong, the skinny body all flaccid and still—

He drew a deep breath.

Foster was walking beside him now, not ahead of him, as though he were a little afraid, and needed reassurance. Indeed the scene had changed. Before and behind them stretched the uphill path, loose with shale and stones. On their right, on a ridge at the foot of the hill, were some quarries, almost deserted, but the more melancholy in the fading afternoon because a little work still continued there, faint sounds came from the gaunt listening chimneys, a stream of water ran and tumbled angrily into a pool below, once and again a black silhouette, like a question mark, appeared against the darkening hill.

It was a little steep here and Foster puffed and blew.

Fenwick hated him the more for that. So thin and spare, and still he could not keep in condition! They stumbled, keeping below the quarry, on the edge of the running water, now green, now a dirty white-grey, pushing their way along the side of the hill.

Their faces were set now towards Helvellyn. It rounded the cup of hills closing in the base and then sprawling to the right.

"There's the tarn!" Fenwick exclaimed—and then added, "The sun's not lasting as long as I had expected. It's growing dark already."

Foster stumbled and caught Fenwick's arm.

"This twilight makes the hills look strange—like living men. I can scarcely see my way."

"We're alone here," Fenwick answered. "Don't you feel the stillness? The men will have left the quarry now and gone home. There is no one in all this place but ourselves. If you watch you will see a strange green light steal down over the hills. It lasts but for a moment, and then it is dark.

"Ah, here is my tarn. Do you know how I love this place, Foster? It seems to belong especially to me, just as much as all your work and your glory and fame and success seem to belong to you. I have this and you have that. Perhaps in the end we are even after all. Yes. . . .

"But I feel as though that piece of water belonged to me and I to it, and as though we should never be separated—yes. . . . Isn't it black?"

"It is one of the deep ones. No one has ever sounded it. Only Helvellyn knows, and one day I fancy that it will take me, too, into its confidence—will whisper its secrets—"

Foster sneezed.

"Very nice. Very beautiful, Fenwick. I like your tarn. Charming. And now let's turn back. That is a difficult walk beneath the quarry. It's chilly, too."

"Do you see that little jetty there?" Fenwick led Foster by the arm. "Someone built that out into the water. He had a boat there, I suppose. Come and look down. From the end of the little jetty it looks so deep and the mountains seem to close round."

Fenwick took Foster's arm and led him to the end of the jetty. Indeed the water looked deep here. Deep and very black. Foster peered down, then he looked up at the hills that did indeed seem to have gathered close around him. He sneezed again.

"I've caught a cold, I am afraid. Let's turn homewards, Fenwick, or we shall never find our way."

"Home then," said Fenwick, and his hands closed about the thin, scraggy neck. For the instant the head half turned and two startled, strangely childish eyes stared; then, with a push that was ludicrously simple, the body was impelled forward, there was a sharp cry, a splash, a stir of something white against the swiftly gathering dusk, again and then again, then far-spreading ripples, then silence.

V

The silence extended. Having enwrapped the tarn, it spread as though with finger on lip to the already quiescent hills. Fenwick shared in the silence. He luxuriated in it. He did not move at all. He stood there looking upon the inky water of the tarn, his arms folded, a man lost in intensest thought. But he was not thinking. He was only conscious of a warm luxurious relief, a sensuous feeling that was not thought at all.

Foster was gone—that tiresome, prating, conceited, self-satisfied fool! Gone, never to return. The tarn assured him of that. It stared back into Fenwick's face approvingly as though it said: "You have done well—a clean and necessary job. We have done it together, you and I. I am proud of you."

He was proud of himself. At last he had done something definite with his life. Thought, eager, active thought, was beginning now to flood his brain. For all these years, he had hung around in this place doing nothing but cherish grievances, weak, backboneless—now at last there was action. He drew himself up and looked at the hills. He was proud—and he was cold. He was shivering. He turned up the collar of his coat. Yes, there was the faint green light that always lingered in the shadows of the hills for a brief moment before darkness came. It was growing late. He had better return.

Shivering now so that his teeth chattered, he started off down the path, and then was aware that he did not wish to leave the tarn. The tarn was friendly; the only friend he had in all the world. As he stumbled along in the dark, this sense of loneliness grew. He was going home to an empty house. There had been a guest in it last night. Who was it? Why, Foster, of course—Foster with his silly laugh and amiable, mediocre eyes. Well, Foster would not be there now. No, he never would be there again.

And suddenly Fenwick started to run. He did not know why, except that, now that he had left the tarn, he was lonely. He wished that he could have stayed there all night, but because he was cold he could not, and now he was running so that he might be at home with the lights and the familiar furniture—and all the things that he knew to reassure him.

As he ran the shale and stones scattered beneath his feet. They made a tit-tattering noise under him, and someone else seemed to be running too. He stopped, and the other runner also stopped. He breathed in the silence. He was hot now. The perspiration was trickling down his cheeks. He could feel a dribble of it down his back inside his shirt. His knees were pounding. His heart was thumping. And all around him, the hills were so amazingly silent, now like indiarubber clouds that you could push in or pull out as you do those indiarubber faces, grey against the night sky of a crystal purple upon whose surface, like the twinkling eyes of boats at sea, stars were now appearing.

His knees steadied, his heart beat less fiercely, and he began to run again.

Suddenly he had turned the corner and was out at the hotel. Its lamps were kindly and reassuring. He walked then quietly along the lake-side path, and had it not been for the certainty that someone was treading behind him he would have been comfortable and at his ease. He stopped once or twice and looked back, and once he stopped and called out "Who's there?" Only the rustling trees answered.

He had the strangest fancy, but his brain was throbbing so fiercely that he could not think, that it was the tarn that was following him, the tarn slipping sliding along the road, being with him so that he should not be lonely. He could almost hear the tarn whisper in his ear: "We did that together, and so I do not wish you to bear all the responsibility yourself. I will stay with you, so that you are not lonely."

He climbed the road towards home, and there were the lights of his house. He heard the gate click behind him as though it were shutting him in. He went into the sitting-room, lighted and ready. There were the books that Foster had admired.

The old woman who looked after him appeared.

"Will you be having some tea, sir?"

"No, thank you, Annie."

"Will the other gentleman be wanting any?"

"No; the other gentleman is away for the night."

"Then there will be only one for supper?"

"Yes, only one for supper."

He sat in the corner of the sofa and fell instantly into a deep slumber.

VI

He woke when the old woman tapped him on the shoulder and told him that supper was served. The room was dark save for the jumping light of two uncertain candles. Those two red candlesticks—how he hated them up there on the mantelpiece! He had always hated them, and now they seemed to him to have something of the quality of Foster's voice—that thin, reedy, piping tone.

He was expecting at every moment that Foster would enter, and yet he knew that he would not. He continued to turn his head towards the door, but it was so dark there that you could not see. The whole room was dark except just there by the fireplace, where the two candlesticks went whining with their miserable twinkling plaint.

He went into the dining-room and sat down to his meal. But he could not eat anything. It was odd—that place by the table where Foster's chair should be. Odd, naked, and made a man feel lonely.

He got up once from the table and went to the window, opened it and looked out. He listened for something. A trickle as of running water, a stir, through the silence, as though some deep pool were filling to the brim. A rustle in the trees, perhaps. An owl hooted. Sharply, as though someone had spoken to him unexpectedly behind his shoulder, he closed the window and looked back, peering under his dark eyebrows into the room.

Later on he went up to bed.

VII

Had he been sleeping, or had he been lying, lazily as one does, half-dozing, half-luxuriously not-thinking? He was wide awake now, utterly awake, and his heart was beating with apprehension. It was as though someone had called him by name. He slept always with his window a little open and the blind up. To-night the moonlight shadowed in sickly fashion the objects in his room. It was not a flood of light nor yet a sharp splash, silvering a square, a circle, throwing the rest into ebony blackness. The light was dim, a little green, perhaps, like the shadow that comes over the hills just before dark.

He stared at the window, and it seemed to him that something moved there. Within, or rather against the green-grey light, something silver-tinted glistened. Fenwick stared. It had the look, exactly, of slipping water.

Slipping water! He listened, his head up, and it seemed to him that from beyond the window he caught the stir of water, not running, but rather welling up and up, gurgling with satisfaction as it filled and filled.

He sat up higher in bed, and then saw that down the wallpaper beneath the window water was undoubtedly trickling. He could see it lurch to the projecting wood of the sill, pause, and then slip, slither down the incline. The odd thing was that it fell so silently.

Beyond the window there was that odd gurgle, but in the room itself absolute silence. Whence could it come? He saw the line of silver rise and fall as the stream on the window-ledge ebbed and flowed.

He must get up and close the window. He drew his legs above the sheets and blankets and looked down.

He shrieked. The floor was covered with a shining film of water. It was rising. As he looked it had covered half the short stumpy legs of the bed. It rose without a wink, a bubble, a break! Over the sill it poured now in a steady flow, but soundless. Fenwick sat back in the bed, the clothes gathered to his chin, his eyes blinking, the Adam's apple throbbing like a throttle in his throat.

But he must do something, he must stop this. The water was now level with the seats of the chairs, but still was soundless. Could he but reach the door!

He put down his naked foot, then cried again. The water was icy cold. Suddenly, leaning, staring at its dark unbroken sheen, something seemed to push him forward. He fell. His head, his face was under the icy liquid; it seemed adhesive and in the heart of its ice hot like melting wax. He struggled to his feet. The water was breast-high. He screamed again and again. He could see the looking-glass, the row of books, the picture of Dürer's 'Horse,' aloof, impervious. He beat at the water and flakes of it seemed to cling to him like scales of fish, clammy to his touch. He struggled, ploughing his way, towards the door.

The water now was at his neck. Then something had caught him by the ankle. Something held him. He struggled, crying, "Let me go! Let me go! I tell you to let me go! I hate you! I hate you! I will not come down to you! I will not—"

The water covered his mouth. He felt that someone pushed in his eyeballs with bare knuckles. A cold hand reached up and caught his naked thigh.

VIII

In the morning the little maid knocked and, receiving no answer, came in as was her wont, with his shaving water. What she saw made her scream. She ran for the gardener.

They took the body with its staring, protruding eyes, its tongue sticking out between the clenched teeth, and laid it on the bed.

The only sign of disorder was an overturned water-jug. A small pool of water stained the carpet.

It was a lovely morning. A twig of ivy idly, in the little breeze, tapped the pane.

William Cowper
FROM THE TASK

From BOOK ONE: THE SOFA

Oh may I live exempted (while I live
Guiltless of pamper'd appetite obscene,)
From pangs arthritic that infest the toe
Of libertine excess. The Sofa suits
The gouty limb, 'tis true; but gouty limb,
Though on a Sofa, may I never feel:
For I have loved the rural walk through lanes
Of grassy swarth close cropt by nibbling sheep,
And skirted thick with intertexture firm
Of thorny boughs; have loved the rural walk
O'er hills, through valleys, and by rivers' brink,
E'er since a truant boy I pass'd my bounds
To enjoy a ramble on the banks of Thames.
And still remember, nor without regret
Of hours that sorrow since has much endear'd,
How oft, my slice of pocket store consumed,
Still hungering pennyless and far from home,
I fed on scarlet hips and stony haws,
Or blushing crabs, or berries that emboss
The bramble, black as jet, or sloes austere.
Hard fare! but such as boyish appetite
Disdains not, nor the palate undepraved
By culinary arts unsavoury deems.
No Sofa then awaited my return,
Nor Sofa then I needed. Youth repairs
His wasted spirits quickly, by long toil

Incurring short fatigue; and though our years
As life declines, speed rapidly away,
And not a year but pilfers as he goes
Some youthful grace that age would gladly keep,
A tooth or auburn lock, and by degrees
Their length and colour from the locks they spare;
The elastic spring of an unwearied foot
That mounts the stile with ease, or leaps the fence,
That play of lungs inhaling and again
Respiring freely the fresh air, that makes
Swift pace or steep ascent no toil to me,
Mine have not pilfer'd yet; nor yet impair'd
My relish of fair prospect; scenes that soothed
Or charm'd me young, no longer young, I find
Still soothing and of power to charm me still.
And witness, dear companion of my walks,
Whose arm this twentieth winter I perceive
Fast lock'd in mine, with pleasure such as love
Confirm'd by long experience of thy worth
And well-tried virtues could alone inspire,—
Witness a joy that thou hast doubled long.
Thou knowest my praise of nature most sincere,
And that my raptures are not conjured up
To serve occasions of poetic pomp,
But genuine, and art partner of them all.
How oft upon yon eminence our pace
Has slacken'd to a pause, and we have borne
The ruffling wind scarce conscious that it blew,
While admiration feeding at the eye,
And still unsated, dwelt upon the scene.
Thence with what pleasure have we just discern'd
The distant plough slow-moving, and beside
His labouring team, that swerved not from the track,
The sturdy swain diminish'd to a boy!
Here Ouse, slow winding through a level plain

Of spacious meads with cattle sprinkled o'er,
Conducts the eye along his sinuous course
Delighted. There, fast rooted in his bank
Stand, never overlook'd, our favourite elms
That screen the herdsman's solitary hut;
While far beyond and overthwart the stream
That as with molten glass inlays the vale,
The sloping land recedes into the clouds;
Displaying on its varied side the grace
Of hedge-row beauties numberless, square tower,
Tall spire, from which the sound of cheerful bells
Just undulates upon the listening ear;
Groves, heaths, and smoking villages remote.
Scenes must be beautiful which daily view'd
Please daily, and whose novelty survives
Long knowledge and the scrutiny of years.
Praise justly due to those that I describe.
       Nor rural sights alone, but rural sounds
Exhilarate the spirit, and restore
The tone of languid Nature. Mighty winds
That sweep the skirt of some far-spreading wood
Of ancient growth, make music not unlike
The dash of ocean on his winding shore,
And lull the spirit while they fill the mind,
Unnumber'd branches waving in the blast,
And all their leaves fast fluttering, all at once.
Nor less composure waits upon the roar
Of distant floods, or on the softer voice
Of neighbouring fountain, or of rills that slip
Through the cleft rock, and chiming as they fall
Upon loose pebbles, lose themselves at length
In matted grass, that with a livelier green
Betrays the secret of their silent course.
Nature inanimate employs sweet sounds,
But animated Nature sweeter still

To soothe and satisfy the human ear.
Ten thousand warblers cheer the day, and one
The livelong night: nor these alone whose notes
Nice-finger'd art must emulate in vain,
But cawing rooks, and kites that swim sublime
In still repeated circles, screaming loud,
The jay, the pie, and even the boding owl
That hails the rising moon, have charms for me.
Sounds inharmonious in themselves and harsh,
Yet heard in scenes where peace for ever reigns,
And only there, please highly for their sake.

      Peace to the artist, whose ingenious thought
Devised the weather-house, that useful toy!
Fearless of humid air and gathering rains
Forth steps the man, an emblem of myself;
More delicate his timorous mate retires.
When Winter soaks the fields, and female feet
Too weak to struggle with tenacious clay,
Or ford the rivulets, are best at home,
The task of new discoveries falls on me.
At such a season and with such a charge
Once went I forth, and found, till then unknown,
A cottage, whither oft we since repair:
'Tis perch'd upon the green-hill top, but close
Environ'd with a ring of branching elms
That overhang the thatch, itself unseen,
Peeps at the vale below; so thick beset
With foliage of such dark redundant growth,
I call'd the low-roof'd lodge the peasant's nest.
And hidden as it is, and far remote
From such unpleasing sounds as haunt the ear
In village or in town, the bay of curs
Incessant, clinking hammers, grinding wheels,
And infants clamorous whether pleased or pain'd,
Oft have I wish'd the peaceful covert mine.

Here, I have said, at least I should possess
The poet's treasure, silence, and indulge
The dreams of fancy, tranquil and secure.
Vain thought! the dweller in that still retreat
Dearly obtains the refuge it affords.
Its elevated site forbids the wretch
To drink sweet waters of the crystal well;
He dips his bowl into the weedy ditch,
And heavy-laden brings his beverage home,
Far-fetch'd and little worth; nor seldom waits,
Dependent on the baker's punctual call,
To hear his creaking panniers at the door,
Angry and sad, and his last crust consumed.
So farewell envy of the peasant's nest.
If solitude make scant the means of life,
Society for me! Thou seeming sweet,
Be still a pleasing object in my view,
My visit still, but never mine abode.

      Not distant far, a length of colonnade
Invites us: Monument of ancient taste,
Now scorn'd, but worthy of a better fate.
Our fathers knew the value of a screen
From sultry suns, and in their shaded walks
And long-protracted bowers, enjoy'd at noon
The gloom and coolness of declining day.
We bear our shades about us; self-deprived
Of other screen, the thin umbrella spread,
And range an Indian waste without a tree.
Thanks to Benevolus; he spares me yet
These chestnuts ranged in corresponding lines,
And though himself so polish'd, still reprieves
The obsolete prolixity of shade.

Descending now (but cautious, lest too fast,)
A sudden steep, upon a rustic bridge

We pass a gulf in which the willows dip
Their pendent boughs, stooping as if to drink.
Hence ancle-deep in moss and flowery thyme
We mount again, and feel at every step
Our foot half sunk in hillocks green and soft,
Raised by the mole, the miner of the soil.
He not unlike the great ones of mankind,
Disfigures earth, and plotting in the dark
Toils much to earn a monumental pile,
That may record the mischiefs he has done.
  The summit gain'd, behold the proud alcove
That crowns it! yet not all its pride secures
The grand retreat from injuries impress'd
By rural carvers, who with knives deface
The panels, leaving an obscure rude name
In characters uncouth, and spelt amiss.
So strong the zeal to immortalize himself
Beats in the breast of man, that even a few
Few transient years won from the abyss abhorr'd
Of blank oblivion, seem a glorious prize,
And even to a clown. Now roves the eye,
And posted on this speculative height
Exults in its command. The sheep-fold here
Pours out its fleecy tenants o'er the glebe.
At first, progressive as a stream, they seek
The middle field; but scatter'd by degrees
Each to his choice, soon whiten all the land.
There, from the sun-burnt hay-field homeward creeps
The loaded wain, while lighten'd of its charge
The wain that meets it passes swiftly by,
The boorish driver leaning o'er his team
Vociferous, and impatient of delay.
Nor less attractive is the woodland scene,
Diversified with trees of every growth
Alike yet various. Here the grey smooth trunks

Of ash, or lime, or beech, distinctly shine,
Within the twilight of their distant shades;
There lost behind a rising ground, the wood
Seems sunk, and shorten'd to its topmost boughs.
No tree in all the grove but has its charms,
Though each its hue peculiar; paler some,
And of a wannish grey; the willow such
And poplar, that with silver lines his leaf,
And ash far-stretching his umbrageous arm;
Of deeper green the elm; and deeper still,
Lord of the woods, the long-surviving oak.
Some glossy-leaved and shining in the sun,
The maple, and the beech of oily nuts
Prolific, and the lime at dewy eve
Diffusing odours: nor unnoted pass
The sycamore, capricious in attire,
Now green, now tawny, and ere autumn yet
Have changed the woods, in scarlet honours bright.
O'er these, but far beyond, (a spacious map
Of hill and valley interposed between,)
The Ouse, dividing the well-water'd land,
Now glitters in the sun, and now retires,
As bashful, yet impatient to be seen.
    Hence the declivity is sharp and short,
And such the re-ascent; between them weeps
A little Naiad her impoverish'd urn
All summer long, which winter fills again.
The folded gates would bar my progress now,
But that the Lord of this enclosed demesne,
Communicative of the good he owns,
Admits me to a share: the guiltless eye
Commits no wrong, nor wastes what it enjoys.
Refreshing change! where now the blazing sun?
By short transition we have lost his glare,
And stepp'd at once into a cooler clime.

Ye fallen avenues! once more I mourn
Your fate unmerited, once more rejoice
That yet a remnant of your race survives.
How airy and how light the graceful arch,
Yet aweful as the consecrated roof
Reechoing pious anthems! while beneath
The chequer'd earth seems restless as a flood
Brush'd by the wind. So sportive is the light
Shot through the boughs, it dances as they dance,
Shadow and sunshine intermingling quick,
And darkening and enlightening, as the leaves
Play wanton, every moment, every spot.
     And now with nerves new-braced and spirits cheer'd
We tread the wilderness, whose well-roll'd walks
With curvature of slow and easy sweep,—
Deception innocent,—give ample space
To narrow bounds. The grove receives us next;
Between the upright shafts of whose tall elms
We may discern the thresher at his task.
Thump after thump, resounds the constant flail,
That seems to swing uncertain, and yet falls
Full on the destined ear. Wide flies the chaff,
The rustling straw sends up a frequent mist
Of atoms sparkling in the noon-day beam.
Come hither, ye that press your beds of down
And sleep not,—see him sweating o'er his bread
Before he eats it.—'Tis the primal curse,
But soften'd into mercy; made the pledge
Of cheerful days, and nights without a groan.
     By ceaseless action, all that is subsists.
Constant rotation of the unwearied wheel
That nature rides upon, maintains her health,
Her beauty, her fertility. She dreads
An instant's pause, and lives but while she moves.
Its own revolvency upholds the world.

Winds from all quarters agitate the air,
And fit the limpid element for use,
Else noxious: oceans, rivers, lakes, and streams
All feel the freshening impulse, and are cleansed
By restless undulation. Even the oak
Thrives by the rude concussion of the storm;
He seems indeed indignant, and to feel
The impression of the blast with proud disdain,
Frowning as if in his unconscious arm
He held the thunder. But the monarch owes
His firm stability to what he scorns,
More fixt below, the more disturb'd above.
The law by which all creatures else are bound,
Binds man the lord of all. Himself derives
No mean advantage from a kindred cause,
From strenuous toil his hours of sweetest ease.
The sedentary stretch their lazy length
When custom bids, but no refreshment find,
For none they need: the languid eye, the cheek
Deserted of its bloom, the flaccid, shrunk,
And wither'd muscle, and the vapid soul,
Reproach their owner with that love of rest
To which he forfeits even the rest he loves.
Not such the alert and active. Measure life
By its true worth, the comforts it affords,
And theirs alone seems worthy of the name.
Good health, and its associate in the most,
Good temper; spirits prompt to undertake,
And not soon spent, though in an arduous task;
The powers of fancy and strong thought are theirs;
Even age itself seems privileged in them
With clear exemption from its own defects.
A sparkling eye beneath a wrinkled front
The veteran shows, and gracing a grey beard
With youthful smiles, descends towards the grave

Sprightly, and old almost without decay.

      Like a coy maiden, ease, when courted most,
Farthest retires,—an idol, at whose shrine
Who oftenest sacrifice are favour'd least.
The love of Nature, and the scenes she draws
Is Nature's dictate. Strange! there should be found
Who self-imprison'd in their proud saloons,
Renounce the odours of the open field
For the unscented fictions of the loom;
Who satisfied with only pencil'd scenes,
Prefer to the performance of a God
The inferior wonders of an artist's hand.
Lovely indeed the mimic works of art,
But Nature's works far lovelier I admire—
None more admires the painter's magic skill,
Who shows me that which I shall never see,
Conveys a distant country into mine,
And throws Italian light on English walls.
But imitative strokes can do no more
Than please the eye, sweet Nature every sense.
The air salubrious of her lofty hills,
The cheering fragrance of her dewy vales
And music of her woods,—no works of man
May rival these; these all bespeak a power
Peculiar, and exclusively her own.
Beneath the open sky she spreads the feast;
'Tis free to all,—'tis every day renew'd,
Who scorns it, starves deservedly at home.
He does not scorn it, who imprison'd long
In some unwholesome dungeon, and a prey
To sallow sickness, which the vapours dank
And clammy of his dark abode have bred,
Escapes at last to liberty and light.
His cheek recovers soon its healthful hue,
His eye relumines its extinguish'd fires,

He walks, he leaps, he runs,—is wing'd with joy,
And riots in the sweets of every breeze.
He does not scorn it, who has long endured
A fever's agonies, and fed on drugs.
Nor yet the mariner, his blood inflamed
With acrid salts; his very heart athirst
To gaze at Nature in her green array.
Upon the ship's tall side he stands, possess'd
With visions prompted by intense desire;
Fair fields appear below, such as he left
Far distant, such as he would die to find,—
He seeks them headlong, and is seen no more.

Patiann Rogers
THERE IS A WAY TO WALK ON WATER

Over the elusive, blue salt-surface easily,
Barefoot, and without surprise—there is a way
To walk far above the tops of volcanic
Scarps and mantle rocks, towering seamounts
Rising in peaks and rifts from the ocean floor,
Over the deep black flow of that distant
Bottom as if one walked studiously
And gracefully on a wire of time
Above eternal night, never touching
Fossil reef corals or the shells of leatherbacks,
Naked gobies or the crusts of sea urchins.

There is a way to walk on water,
And it has something to do with the feel
Of the silken waves sliding continuously
And carefully against the inner arches
Of the feet; and something to do
With what the empty hands, open above
The weed-blown current and chasm
Of that possible fall, hold to tightly;
Something to do with how clearly
And simply one can imagine a silver scatter
Of migrating petrels flying through the body
During that instant, gliding with their white
Wings spread through the cartilage of throat
And breast, across the vast dome of the skull,
How distinctly one can hear them calling singly
And together inside the lungs, sailing straight

Through the spine as if they themselves believed
That bone and moment were passageways
Of equal accessibility.

Buoyant and inconsequential, as serious,
As exact as stone, that old motion of the body,
That visible stride of the soul, when the measured
Placing of each toe, the perfect justice
Of the feet, seems a sublimity of event,
A spatial exaltation—to be able to walk
Over water like that has something to do
With the way, like a rain-filled wind coming
Again to dry grasses on a prairie, all
Of these possibilities are remembered at once,
And the way, like many small blind mouths
Taking drink in their dark sleep,
All of these powers are discovered,
Complete and accomplished
And present from the beginning.

Samuel Taylor Coleridge
THIS LIME-TREE BOWER MY PRISON

Well, they are gone, and here must I remain,
This lime-tree bower my prison! I have lost
Beauties and feelings, such as would have been
Most sweet to my remembrance even when age
Had dimm'd mine eyes to blindness! They, meanwhile,
Friends, whom I never more may meet again,
On springy heath, along the hill-top edge,
Wander in gladness, and wind down, perchance,
To that still roaring dell, of which I told;
The roaring dell, o'erwooded, narrow, deep,
And only speckled by the mid-day sun;
Where its slim trunk the ash from rock to rock
Flings arching like a bridge;—that branchless ash,
Unsunn'd and damp, whose few poor yellow leaves
Ne'er tremble in the gale, yet tremble still,
Fann'd by the water-fall! and there my friends
Behold the dark green file of long lank weeds,
That all at once (a most fantastic sight!)
Still nod and drip beneath the dripping edge
Of the blue clay-stone.

                    Now, my friends emerge
Beneath the wide wide Heaven—and view again
The many-steepled tract magnificent
Of hilly fields and meadows, and the sea,
With some fair bark, perhaps, whose sails light up
The slip of smooth clear blue betwixt two Isles
Of purple shadow! Yes! they wander on

In gladness all; but thou, methinks, most glad,
My gentle-hearted Charles! for thou hast pined
And hunger'd after Nature, many a year,
In the great City pent, winning thy way
With sad yet patient soul, through evil and pain
And strange calamity! Ah! slowly sink
Behind the western ridge, thou glorious Sun!
Shine in the slant beams of the sinking orb,
Ye purple heath-flowers! richlier burn, ye clouds!
Live in the yellow light, ye distant groves!
And kindle, thou blue Ocean! So my friend
Struck with deep joy may stand, as I have stood,
Silent with swimming sense; yea, gazing round
On the wide landscape, gaze till all doth seem
Less gross than bodily; and of such hues
As veil the Almighty Spirit, when yet he makes
Spirits perceive his presence.

                            A delight
Comes sudden on my heart, and I am glad
As I myself were there! Nor in this bower,
This little lime-tree bower, have I not mark'd
Much that has sooth'd me. Pale beneath the blaze
Hung the transparent foliage; and I watch'd
Some broad and sunny leaf, and lov'd to see
The shadow of the leaf and stem above
Dappling its sunshine! And that walnut-tree
Was richly ting'd, and a deep radiance lay
Full on the ancient ivy, which usurps
Those fronting elms, and now, with blackest mass
Makes their dark branches gleam a lighter hue
Through the late twilight: and though now the bat
Wheels silent by, and not a swallow twitters,
Yet still the solitary humble-bee
Sings in the bean-flower! Henceforth I shall know

That Nature ne'er deserts the wise and pure;
No plot so narrow, be but Nature there,
No waste so vacant, but may well employ
Each faculty of sense, and keep the heart
Awake to Love and Beauty! and sometimes
'Tis well to be bereft of promis'd good,
That we may lift the soul, and contemplate
With lively joy the joys we cannot share.
My gentle-hearted Charles! when the last rook
Beat its straight path along the dusky air
Homewards, I blest it! deeming its black wing
(Now a dim speck, now vanishing in light)
Had cross'd the mighty Orb's dilated glory,
While thou stood'st gazing; or, when all was still,
Flew creeking o'er thy head, and had a charm
For thee, my gentle-hearted Charles, to whom
No sound is dissonant which tells of Life.

John Gay
FROM TRIVIA; OR, THE ART OF WALKING THE STREETS OF LONDON

From BOOK III
Of Walking the Streets by Night

O Trivia, Goddess, leave these low abodes,
And traverse o'er the wide ethereal roads,
Celestial Queen, put on thy robes of light,
Now Cynthia nam'd, fair regent of the Night.
At sight of thee the villain sheaths his sword,
Nor scales the wall, to steal the wealthy hoard.
O may thy silver lamp from heav'n's high bow'r
Direct my footsteps in the midnight hour!

When night first bids the twinkling stars appear,
Or with her cloudy vest inwraps the air,
Then swarms the busie street; with caution tread,
Where the shop-windows falling threat thy head;
Now lab'rers home return, and join their strength
To bear the tott'ring plank, or ladder's length;
Still fix thy eyes intent upon the throng,
And as the passes open, wind along.

Where the fair columns of St. Clement stand,
Whose straiten'd bounds encroach upon the Strand;
Where the low penthouse bows the walker's head,
And the rough pavement wounds the yielding tread;
Where not a post protects the narrow space,
And strung in twines, combs dangle in thy face;

Summon at once thy courage, rouze thy care,
Stand firm, look back, be resolute, beware.
Forth issuing from steep lanes, the collier's steeds
Drag the black load; another cart succeeds,
Team follows team, crouds heap'd on crouds appear,
And wait impatient, 'till the road grow clear.
Now all the pavement sounds with trampling feet,
And the mixt hurry barricades the street.
Entangled here, the waggon's lengthen'd team
Cracks the tough harness; here a pond'rous beam
Lies over-turn'd athwart; for slaughter fed
Here lowing bullocks raise their horned head.
Now oaths grow loud, with coaches coaches jar,
And the smart blow provokes the sturdy war;
From the high box they whirl the thong around,
And with the twining lash their shins resound:
Their rage ferments, more dang'rous wounds they try,
And the blood gushes down their painful eye.
And now on foot the frowning warriors light,
And with their pond'rous fists renew the fight;
Blow answers blow, their cheeks are smear'd with blood,
'Till down they fall, and grappling roll in mud.
So when two boars, in wild Ytene bred,
Or on Westphalia's fatt'ning chest-nuts fed,
Gnash their sharp tusks, and rous'd with equal fire,
Dispute the reign of some luxurious mire;
In the black flood they wallow o'er and o'er,
'Till their arm'd jaws distil with foam and gore.

Where the mob gathers, swiftly shoot along,
Nor idly mingle in the noisy throng.
Lur'd by the silver hilt, amid the swarm,
The subtil artist will thy side disarm.
Nor is thy flaxen wigg with safety worn;
High on the shoulder, in a basket born,
Lurks the sly boy; whose hand to rapine bred,

Plucks off the curling honours of thy head.
Here dives the skulking thief with practis'd slight,
And unfelt fingers make thy pocket light.
Where's now thy watch, with all its trinkets, flown?
And thy late snuff-box is no more thy own.
But lo! his bolder theft some tradesman spies,
Swift from his prey the scudding lurcher flies;
Dext'rous he 'scapes the coach with nimble bounds,
Whilst ev'ry honest tongue 'stop thief' resounds.
So speeds the wily fox, alarm'd by fear,
Who lately filch'd the turkey's callow care;
Hounds following hounds grow louder as he flies,
And injur'd tenants joyn the hunter's cries.
Breathless he stumbling falls: Ill-fated boy!
Why did not honest work thy youth employ?
Seiz'd by rough hands, he's dragg'd amid the rout,
And stretch'd beneath the pump's incessant spout:
Or plung'd in miry ponds, he gasping lies,
Mud choaks his mouth, and plaisters o'er his eyes.

Let not the ballad-singer's shrilling strain
Amid the swarm thy list'ning ear detain:
Guard well thy pocket; for these Syrens stand
To aid the labours of the diving hand;
Confed'rate in the cheat, they draw the throng,
And cambrick handkerchiefs reward the song.
But soon as coach or cart drives rattling on,
The rabble part, in shoals they backward run.
So Jove's loud bolts the mingled war divide,
And Greece and Troy retreat on either side.

If the rude throng pour on with furious pace,
And hap to break thee from a friend's embrace,
Stop short; nor struggle through the croud in vain,
But watch with careful eye the passing train.
Yet I (perhaps too fond) if chance the tide

Tumultuous bear my partner from my side,
Impatient venture back; despising harm,
I force my passage where the thickest swarm.
Thus his lost bride the Trojan sought in vain
Through night, and arms, and flames, and hills of slain.
Thus Nisus wander'd o'er the pathless grove,
To find the brave companion of his love,
The pathless grove in vain he wanders o'er:
Euryalus, alas! is now no more.

That walker, who regardless of his pace,
Turns oft' to pore upon the damsel's face,
From side to side by thrusting elbows tost,
Shall strike his aking breast against the post;
Or water, dash'd from fishy stalls, shall stain
His hapless coat with spirts of scaly rain.
But if unwarily he chance to stray,
Where twirling turnstiles intercept the way,
The thwarting passenger shall force them round,
And beat the wretch half breathless to the ground.

Let constant vigilance thy footsteps guide,
And wary circumspection guard thy side;
Then shalt thou walk unharm'd the dang'rous night,
Nor need th' officious link-boy's smoaky light.
Thou never wilt attempt to cross the road,
Where alehouse benches rest the porter's load,
Grievous to heedless shins; no barrow's wheel,
That bruises oft' the truant school-boy's heel,
Behind thee rolling, with insidious pace,
Shall mark thy stocking with a miry trace.
Let not thy vent'rous steps approach too nigh,
Where gaping wide, low steepy cellars lie;
Should thy shoe wrench aside, down, down you fall,
And overturn the scolding huckster's stall,
The scolding huckster shall not o'er thee moan,

But pence exact for nuts and pears o'erthrown.

Though you through cleanlier allies wind by day,
To shun the hurries of the publick way,
Yet ne'er to those dark paths by night retire;
Mind only safety, and contemn the mire.
Then no impervious courts thy haste detain,
Nor sneering ale-wives bid thee turn again.

Where Lincoln's-Inn, wide space, is rail'd around,
Cross not with vent'rous step; there oft' is found
The lurking thief, who while the day-light shone,
Made the walls eccho with his begging tone:
That crutch which late compassion mov'd, shall wound
Thy bleeding head, and fell thee to the ground.
Though thou art tempted by the link-man's call,
Yet trust him not along the lonely wall;
In the mid-way he'll quench the flaming brand,
And share the booty with the pilf'ring band.
Still keep the publick streets, where oily rays
Shot from the crystal lamp, o'erspread the ways.

Happy Augusta! law-defended town!
Here no dark lanthorns shade the villain's frown;
No Spanish jealousies thy lanes infest,
Nor Roman vengeance stabs th' unwary breast;
Here tyranny ne'er lifts her purple hand,
But liberty and justice guard the land;
No bravos here profess the bloody trade,
Nor is the church the murd'rer's refuge made.

Let not the chairman, with assuming stride,
Press near the wall, and rudely thrust thy side:
The laws have set him bounds; his servile feet
Should ne'er encroach where posts defend the street.

Yet who the footman's arrogance can quell,
Whose flambeau gilds the sashes of Pell-mell,
When in long rank a train of torches flame,
To light the midnight visits of the dame?
Others, perhaps, by happier guidance led,
May where the chairman rests, with safety tread;
Whene'er I pass, their poles unseen below,
Make my knee tremble with the jarring blow.

If wheels bar up the road, where streets are crost,
With gentle words the coachman's ear accost:
He ne'er the threat, or harsh command obeys,
But with contempt the spatter'd shoe surveys.
Now man with utmost fortitude thy soul,
To cross the way where carts and coaches roll;
Yet do not in thy hardy skill confide,
Nor rashly risque the kennel's spacious stride;
Stay till afar the distant wheel you hear,
Like dying thunder in the breaking air;
Thy foot will slide upon the miry stone,
And passing coaches crush thy tortur'd bone,
Or wheels enclose the road; on either hand
Pent round with perils, in the midst you stand,
And call for aid in vain; the coachman swears,
And car-men drive, unmindful of thy prayers.
Where wilt thou turn? ah! whither wilt thou fly?
On ev'ry side the pressing spokes are nigh.
So sailors, while Carybdis' gulph they shun,
Amaz'd, on Scylla's craggy dangers run.

Be sure observe where brown Ostrea stands,
Who boasts her shelly ware from Wallfleet sands;
There may'st thou pass, with safe unmiry feet,
Where the rais'd pavement leads athwart the street.
If where Fleet-ditch with muddy current flows,

You chance to roam; where oyster-tubs in rows
Are rang'd beside the posts; there stay thy haste,
And with the sav'ry fish indulge thy taste:
The damsel's knife the gaping shell commands,
While the salt liquor streams between her hands.

The man had sure a palate cover'd o'er
With brass or steel, that on the rocky shore
First broke the oozy oyster's pearly coat,
And risqu'd the living morsel down his throat.
What will not lux'ry taste? Earth, sea, and air
Are daily ransack'd for the bill of fare.
Blood stuff'd in skins is British Christians' food,
And France robs marshes of the croaking brood;
Spongy morells in strong ragousts are found,
And in the soupe the slimy snail is drown'd.

When from high spouts the dashing torrents fall,
Ever be watchful to maintain the wall;
For should'st thou quit thy ground, the rushing throng
Will with impetuous fury drive along;
All press to gain those honours thou hast lost,
And rudely shove thee far without the post.
Then to retrieve the shed you strive in vain,
Draggled all o'er, and soak'd in floods of rain.
Yet rather bear the show'r, and toils of mud,
Than in the doubtful quarrel risque thy blood.
O think on Oedipus' detested state,
And by his woes be warn'd to shun thy fate.

Where three roads join'd, he met his sire unknown;
(Unhappy sire, but more unhappy son!)
Each claim'd the way, their swords the strife decide,
The hoary monarch fell, he groan'd and dy'd!
Hence sprung the fatal plague that thin'd thy reign,

Thy cursed incest! and thy children slain!
Hence wert thou doom'd in endless night to stray
Through Theban streets, and cheerless groap thy way.

Contemplate, mortal, on thy fleeting years;
See, with black train the funeral pomp appears!
Whether some heir attends in sable state,
And mourns with outward grief a parent's fate;
Or the fair virgin, nipt in beauty's bloom,
A croud of lovers follow to her tomb.
Why is the herse with 'scutcheons blazon'd round,
And with the nodding plume of Ostrich crown'd?
No: The dead know it not, nor profit gain;
It only serves to prove the living vain.
How short is life! how frail is human trust!
Is all this pomp for laying dust to dust?

Where the nail'd hoop defends the painted stall,
Brush not thy sweeping skirt too near the wall;
Thy heedless sleeve will drink the colour'd oil,
And spot indelible thy pocket soil.
Has not wise nature strung the legs and feet
With firmest nerves, design'd to walk the street?
Has she not given us hands, to groap aright,
Amidst the frequent dangers of the night?
And think'st thou not the double nostril meant,
To warn from oily woes by previous scent?

Who can the various city frauds recite,
With all the petty rapines of the night?
Who now the Guinea-dropper's bait regards,
Trick'd by the sharper's dice, or juggler's cards?
Why should I warn thee ne'er to join the fray,
Where the sham-quarrel interrupts the way?
Lives there in these our days so soft a clown,

Brav'd by the bully's oaths, or threat'ning frown?
I need not strict enjoyn the pocket's care,
When from the crouded play thou lead'st the fair;
Who has not here, or watch, or snuff-box lost,
Or handkerchiefs that India's shuttle boast?

O! may thy virtue guard thee through the roads
Of Drury's mazy courts, and dark abodes,
The harlots' guileful paths, who nightly stand,
Where Katherine-street descends into the Strand.
Say, vagrant Muse, their wiles and subtil arts,
To lure the strangers unsuspecting hearts;
So shall our youth on healthful sinews tread,
And city cheeks grow warm with rural red.

'Tis she who nightly strowls with saunt'ring pace,
No stubborn stays her yielding shape embrace;
Beneath the lamp her tawdry ribbons glare,
The new-scower'd manteau, and the slattern air;
High-draggled petticoats her travels show,
And hollow cheeks with artful blushes glow;
With flatt'ring sounds she sooths the cred'lous ear,
My noble captain! charmer! love! my dear!
In riding-hood near tavern-doors she plies,
Or muffled pinners hide her livid eyes.
With empty bandbox she delights to range,
And feigns a distant errand from the 'Change;
Nay, she will oft' the Quaker's hood prophane,
And trudge demure the rounds of Drury-lane.
She darts from sarsnet ambush wily leers,
Twitches thy sleeve, or with familiar airs
Her fan will pat thy cheek; these snares disdain,
Nor gaze behind thee, when she turns again.

I knew a yeoman, who for thirst of gain,

To the great city drove from Devon's plain
His num'rous lowing herd; his herds he sold,
And his deep leathern pocket bagg'd with gold;
Drawn by a fraudful nymph, he gaz'd, he sigh'd;
Unmindful of his home, and distant bride,
She leads the willing victim to his doom,
Through winding alleys to her cobweb room.
Thence thro' the street he reels from post to post,
Valiant with wine, nor knows his treasure lost.
The vagrant wretch th' assembled watchmen spies,
He waves his hanger, and their poles defies;
Deep in the Round-house pent, all night he snores,
And the next morn in vain his fate deplores.

Ah hapless swain, unus'd to pains and ills!
Canst thou forego roast-beef for nauseous pills?
How wilt thou lift to Heav'n thy eyes and hands,
When the long scroll the surgeon's fees demands!
Or else (ye Gods avert that worst disgrace)
Thy ruin'd nose falls level with thy face,
Then shall thy wife thy loathsome kiss disdain,
And wholesome neighbours from thy mug refrain.

Yet there are watchmen, who with friendly light
Will teach thy reeling steps to tread aright;
For sixpence will support thy helpless arm,
And home conduct thee, safe from nightly harm;
But if they shake their lanthorns, from afar
To call their breth'ren to confed'rate war
When rakes resist their pow'r; if hapless you
Should chance to wander with the scow'ring crew;
Though fortune yield thee captive, ne'er despair,
But seek the constable's consid'rate ear;
He will reverse the watchman's harsh decree,
Moved by the rhet'rick of a silver fee.

Thus would you gain some fav'rite courtier's word;
Fee not the petty clarks, but bribe my Lord.

Now is the time that rakes their revells keep;
Kindlers of riot, enemies of sleep.
His scatter'd pence the flying Nicker flings,
And with the copper show'r the casement rings.
Who has not heard the Scowrer's midnight fame?
Who has not trembled at the Mohock's name?
Was there a watchman took his hourly rounds,
Safe from their blows, or new-invented wounds?
I pass their desp'rate deeds, and mischiefs done
Where from Snow-hill black steepy torrents run;
How matrons, hoop'd within the hoghead's womb,
Were tumbled furious thence, the rolling tomb
O'er the stones thunders, bounds from side to side.
So Regulus to save his country dy'd.

Where a dim gleam the paly lanthorn throws
O'er the mid pavement, heapy rubbish grows;
Or arched vaults their gaping jaws extend,
Or the dark caves to common-shores descend.
Oft' by the winds extinct the signal lies,
Or smother'd in the glimmering socket dies,
E'er night has half roll'd round her ebon throne;
In the wide gulph the shatter'd coach o'erthrown
Sinks with the snorting steeds; the reins are broke,
And from the crackling axle flies the spoke.
So when fam'd Eddystone's far-shooting ray,
That led the sailor through the stormy way,
Was from its rocky roots by billows torn,
And the high turret in the whirlewind born,
Fleets bulg'd their sides against the craggy land,
And pitchy ruines blacken'd all the strand.

Who then through night would hire the harness'd steed,
And who would choose the rattling wheel for speed?

But hark! distress with screaming voice draws nigh'r,
And wakes the slumb'ring street with cries of fire.
At first a glowing red enwraps the skies,
And born by winds the scatt'ring sparks arise;
From beam to beam the fierce contagion spreads;
The spiry flames now lift aloft their heads,
Through the burst sash a blazing deluge pours,
And splitting tiles descend in rattling show'rs.
Now with thick crouds th' enlighten'd pavement swarms,
The fire-man sweats beneath his crooked arms,
A leathern casque his vent'rous head defends,
Boldly he climbs where thickest smoak ascends;
Mov'd by the mother's streaming eyes and pray'rs,
The helpless infant through the flame he bears,
With no less virtue, than through hostile fire
The Dardan hero bore his aged sire.
See forceful engines spout their levell'd streams,
To quench the blaze that runs along the beams;
The grappling hook plucks rafters from the walls,
And heaps on heaps the smoaky ruine falls.
Blown by strong winds the fiery tempest roars,
Bears down new walls, and pours along the floors;
The Heav'ns are all a-blaze, the face of night
Is cover'd with a sanguine dreadful light:
'Twas such a light involv'd thy tow'rs, O Rome,
The dire presage of mighty Cæsar's doom,
When the sun veil'd in rust his mourning head,
And frightful prodigies the skies o'erspread.
Hark! the drum thunders! far, ye crouds, retire:
Behold! the ready match is tipt with fire,
The nitrous store is laid, the smutty train
With running blaze awakes the barrell'd grain;

Flames sudden wrap the walls; with sullen sound
The shatter'd pile sinks on the smoaky ground.
So when the years shall have revolv'd the date,
Th' inevitable hour of Naples' fate,
Her sapp'd foundations shall with thunders shake,
And heave and toss upon the sulph'rous lake;
Earth's womb at once the fiery flood shall rend,
And in th' abyss her plunging tow'rs descend.

Consider, reader, what fatigues I've known,
The toils, the perils of the wintry town;
What riots seen, what bustling crouds I bor'd,
How oft' I cross'd where carts and coaches roar'd;
Yet shall I bless my labours, if mankind
Their future safety from my dangers find.
Thus the bold traveller, (inur'd to toil,
Whose steps have printed Asia's desert soil,
The barb'rous Arabs haunt; or shiv'ring crost
Dark Greenland's mountains of eternal frost;
Whom providence in length of years restores
To the wish'd harbour of his native shores;)
Sets forth his journals to the publick view,
To caution, by his woes, the wand'ring crew.

And now compleat my gen'rous labours lye,
Finish'd, and ripe for immortality.
Death shall entomb in dust this mould'ring frame,
But never reach th' eternal part, my fame.
When W— and G—, mighty names, are dead;
Or but at Chelsea under custards read;
When Criticks crazy bandboxes repair,
And Tragedies, turn'd rockets, bounce in air;
High-rais'd on Fleet-street posts, consign'd to fame,
This work shall shine, and walkers bless my name.

Adrienne Rich
UPPER BROADWAY

The leafbud straggles forth
toward the frigid light of the airshaft   this is faith
this pale extension of a day
when looking up you know something is changing
winter has turned though the wind is colder
Three streets away a roof collapses onto people
who thought they still had time Time out of mind

I have written so many words
wanting to live inside you
to be of use to you

Now I must write for myself for this blind
woman scratching the pavement with her wand of thought
this slippered crone inching on icy streets
reaching into wire trashbaskets pulling out
what was thrown away and infinitely precious

I look at my hands and see they are still unfinished
I look at the vine and see the leafbud
inching towards life

I look at my face in the glass and see
halfborn woman

Gabriela Mistral
THE USELESS VIGIL

I forgot that your light foot
was transformed into ashes,
and, as during good times,
I ventured to find you
along the path.

I passed through valley,
plain and river;
songs filled me with melancholy.
Afternoon faded,
tumbled its luminous vase.
And you didn't appear!

The sun crumbled its poppy,
charred and lifeless.
A foggy fringe trembled
over the fields.
I was alone!

From a tree,
a whitened branch like an arm,
rustled in the autumn wind.
I was terrified and cried out to you,
"My love, hurry to my side!"

"I hold fear
and I hold onto love.
My love, speed your journey!"

Night thickened around me;
my madness grew.

I forgot—they made you deaf
to my lament;
your deadly dawn,

your heavy hand,
too late, its quest for my hand,
and your wide eyes,
a sovereign inquisition!

Night extended
its bituminous-black pool;
The owl of mystic fortune
fretted the path
with the macabre silk
of its wings.
I will not call out to you again;
your journey has ended.
My naked foot continues its trek;
 your foot remains eternally quiet.

In vain I hold this vigil
along deserted roads.
Your ghost will not come together
in my open arms!

Merle Collins
THE WALK

Faith reached up and unbuttoned the apron at the back. Let it drop to the front. Reached back and loosened the knot at her waist. Pulled off the apron and dropped it on to the barrel behind the door. She slumped on to the bench just inside of the kitchen door. She looked across at the fireside, at the scattered bits of wood, at the ashes cold and grey around the wood. Her eyes moved automatically towards the coal-pot, where a yellow butter-pan rested on partly burnt-out coals. She wondered whether Queen had prepared anything. To tell the truth, she was too tired to really care. She turned and looked at the bucket of water on the dresser, at the two pancups hanging from a nail above it. She took a deep breath, released it and let her head fall forward on to the rough board of the kitchen table.

"Oh God ah tired!" For a few moments, Faith remained like that, letting her body savour what it was like to be sitting down, letting it relax. And then her bottom registered that there was something hard on the bench. Faith's hand found the pebble, removed it. She sat up with a sigh and threw the pebble through the window over the shelf. Faith looked down at the floor. Yes. Queen had scrubbed it. A good child, when she put her mind to it.

Faith leaned back against the brown board of the partition and closed her eyes.

"Queen! Queenie oh! Bring some water give me!"

Queen came running, "Mammie I didn't hear you come, non! And I look out the back window and I see light in the Great House still, and I see a lot of cars go up, so I say they having party, and . . ."

"All right. All right!"

Faith held the pancup with both hands, drinking the water in great gulps.

"Ah! Dat good! You boil de cocoa tea?"

"Yes, Mammie."

"The lady pay me dis evening. I want you to go up for me tomorrow mornin."

Queen sucked her teeth. "Mammie I . . ."

"You what?" Faith sat up, her eyes demanding the response they defied her daughter to make. "Look, child! If you know what good for you, move out of me eyesight, eh! You have to go up for me tomorrow and pay de society, an Cousin Kamay have the little pig mindin so I could turn me hand to something. I want you to pass and see if it drop already. You remember de house where I did show you Cousin Sésé daughter livin?"

"De house wid de green gate and the yellow curtain in the window?"

"So if they change de curtain you won't know de house?"

"Ay! Yes, Mammie, it have a big mammie apple tree in the yard."

"Right. Pass there and tell Cousin Sésé daughter, Miss Ivy, I ask if de message ready already."

"Yes, Mammie."

Faith looked at her daughter standing beside the bucket of water, at her bony, long-legged frame in the baggy dress. She sighed. It would be a long walk, but Queen was used to it. She wished she didn't have to take the child away from school to make these errands, but what with living so far away and not being able to get a job nearer to the family! And she *must* pay the society. If she dropped down tomorrow morning, what would happen to Queen? A person must make sure to put by a little. You never know when you time would come without warning! And if the pig drop now, she could sell one and have enough to at least buy a little bed. And perhaps she might even be able to take out a better susu hand. Anyway, don't count you chickens! Just hope for the best. Just hope!

"Don't drink too much water, Queen. Next thing you know, you playin baby give me an wetting you bed. Is time for you to go an sleep. You have to get up early. You drink the coraile bush for the cold?"

"Yes, Mammie, an I make some bakes and put in de safe."

"Good. That good. You a real help to me, yes. I don't know what I would do without you, child! Take de small lamp an go inside and sleep. Leave de masanto here for me. What light you sit down inside there with? You have a candle?"

"No, Mammie, I was just sitting down looking out of the back window at the Great House lights."

"Sitting down in the dark, Queen? Why you didn't take the small lamp all the time?"

"Was only for a little while, yes, Mammie, after I finish clean up the kitchen."

"All right, go on! Go on and get ready for bed!"

Queen took the lamp and walked out of the kitchen door. For just a moment she glanced to the left, at the quiet, dark outline of coconut trees. But she didn't like the way the coconut trees rustled, and besides you could never trust a sudden breeze not to put the lamplight out.

Queen climbed the two wooden steps into the house, placed the lamp on the shelf and prepared for bed. She was thinking of the following morning's walk as she pulled the pile of bedding from under the sofa in the corner and spread it out. Queen did not like having to walk all the way to River Sallee. The road was long. She was always afraid to walk that long road. Queen stood for a long while staring at the lamp. She looked at the partition above the lamp, at the picture which had written on it, *God Save Our Gracious King*. Thrown over the top of this picture was her mother's chaplet, the cross resting on the king's forehead. Queen wasn't really *seeing* the picture. She was thinking. Wondering who and who was going to make that walk to River Sallee with her tomorrow morning. Who else was going up? In her hand was the old, torn dress that her mother no longer wore and which she was about to spread out on the floor over the other things already there Queen walked to the door, her dress band trailing. She had already undone the fastener at the back, and the dress was drooping, baring one bony shoulder.

"Mammie! Cousin Liza goin up tomorrow too?"

"Yes. She goin to call for you early in the morning. You say you prayers yet?"

"No Mammie. I goin an say it now."

Queen changed quickly, knelt down, bent her forehead to touch the sofa, and prayed aloud: "Gentle Jesus meek and mild, look upon a little child!"

She lifted her head and looked at the crucifix over the bed. "Papa God, help me to grow up into a big strong girl for me please. God don't let me die tonight or any other night please. Bless Mammie and Cousin Dinah and Maisie and Mark. Make the walk tomorrow not hard please and don't let me and Cousin Liza meet anything in the road. Bless Cousin Liza too and let me have a lot a lot of money when I get big please God. Amen."

Still on her knees, Queen lifted her head.

"Good-night, Mammie."

"Good-night, chile. Turn down de lamp low."

"You not goin an sleep now, Mammie?"

"Yes. I just takin a little rest fus."

"Well come and rest inside here, non, Mammie."

"Queenie hush you mouth an sleep now. You pray already. Stop talkin like dat after you pray."

About an hour later, Faith, having eaten some of the bake from the safe and allowed the day's weariness to seep from her body through the boards to the still, hot air outside, walked heavily up the two board steps and into the house. There was some noise as she passed briefly through the watching darkness; a cat scuttling, perhaps, a dog scratching, a frog hopping by. Faith didn't look around. She hardly heard them. The sounds of darkness were always with her. Nothing strange.

Her young Queen was fast asleep, mouth slightly open, left hand thrown wide and resting on the floor outside the bedding, the cover partly twisted around her waist. The mother stood staring for a moment, then stooped to straighten the piece of bedding which served as a cover and pulled it up over her daughter's body. She turned to the sofa, then sank to her knees and bowed her head. Faith spoke no words aloud. She talked silently to the Lord. Her last waking thoughts were, Today is the madam party. I wonder if Mr Mark suit . . .

When Cousin Liza pounded at the door on that February morning in 1931, it was still the time of day when everyone whispered. Dark and cold in the kind of way it never was when the sun came up. It was still the time that the trees claimed as their own as they whispered secrets against the sky. They whispered something when Cousin Liza knocked, and she looked around nervously, but they became silent then.

The walk from St David's to River Sallee was a long and arduous one. It was best started early. Queen was still half-asleep when they left. But the way Cousin Liza walked, sleep didn't stay around for long. It departed with a frown and an irritated yawn. Wide awake after the first few minutes, Queen pushed the straw hat more firmly on to her head, held the cloth bag securely on her shoulder, and kept running to keep up.

Cousin Liza had planned to start at five A.M. She must have made a mistake, though. Day was a long time coming, and the trees and the shadows and the frogs shouting in the drains kept insisting that it was still their time. They had been walking for more than two hours when the first glimmers of dawn appeared. At one time they had passed a house in which a light burned brightly. The man inside may have seen them, for the door was open. Into the darkness he shouted, "Wey dis two woman goin at this hour?" and his feet pounded on the floor as though he were coming out to get them. If she had known who he was, Cousin Liza wouldn't be afraid, but you never knew with people who were up that late. They could be doing all sorts of things with the supernatural. So Cousin Liza pulled Queen and they pelted off down the road, feet flying on the broken pavement. After this, Queen was afraid, for she realized that Cousin Liza, too, talked with fear.

At one point, when they got to a place where the road forked in three directions, Queen did not find it strange to see a cock standing in the middle of the crossroads. She was accustomed to fowls. It was only when she felt Cousin Liza jerk her towards the drain that she froze. They passed in the drain at the side of the road and walked without looking back. Cousin Liza did not have to tell Queen it would be dangerous to look back. She *knew!* Queen's whole body was heart. It pounded with a painful thump that resounded in her steps. Her bare feet felt neither the stones in the road nor the effect of the miles. Suspended in a twilight between conscious thought and puppetry, she knew neither where she was nor where she was going to. And worse was yet to come.

They were making their way through a track in Hope, St Andrew's, which could cut down on the distance to Grenville town, when Queen pulled convulsively on Cousin Liza's hand. Liza's twenty-eight years on what she knew of earth had not given her the fearlessness that Queen expected her to possess. Queen stood, one hand now on top of the straw hat the brim of which framed her round face, the thick black plaits sticking out on both sides, the other hand lifted towards the distance. Liza froze. With a taut, tense movement she boxed down the child's shaking finger.

"Don't point," she whispered hoarsely. "Bite you finger," she remembered to add.

On the hill next to the gravestone, something moved. No house was in sight. Above the watching women, the branches of the trees leaned across and linked leaves, touching each other caressingly in the stillness of the morning. The thing moved again. A pale light from a wandering, waning moon flashed across it and the thing bent towards them, beckoning, encouraging them forward. Queen's arms were thrown around Liza and she clung tightly, mouth open, the breath pushed from her throat to her lips in audible sobs, eyes wide with terror. Liza, body and hands hard with fear, held on to the child. She uttered no prayer with her lips, none in her heart. Her whole body was a throbbing prayer. Papa God! Papa God!

Whatever it was was quiet now. Still, no longer beckoning. The leaves above, too, had stopped their furtive caressing. Liza's feet moved. One quiet dragging step. Two, the left foot following because it couldn't go off on its own in a different direction. T-h-r-ee. Queen's body, with no will or separate identity of its own, did whatever Liza's did. The thing bent towards them. Queen screamed. With sudden decision, Liza dragged Queen along the edge of the track. And as this living fear drew level with the taunting thing above, it stopped in unbelief.

"Jesus!" said Cousin Liza. "Jesus!"

The plantain leaf bowed again.

Queen, sobbing now with the release of terror, clung to Cousin Liza's hand and was dragged along the track. Her destination was daylight. It was only when the sky lightened and she could hear cocks crowing and see people moving about in the yards that she became once more a conscious being. She started to feel tired and told Cousin Liza that she wanted to rest.

They had been walking for seven hours and were in Paradise with the sun blazing down upon their heads when the bus from St David's passed them on its way to Sauteurs. Queen ate her coconut-drops and stretched out her tongue at the people looking back from the back seat of the bus. Years later, an older Queen learnt that the threepence she and Cousin Liza had spent to buy things to eat along the way could have paid a bus fare. Even though she had known then, the knowledge would have been of little use. Faith would have called her damn lazy if she had suggested going by bus.

"Liza, girl, you must be tired. How you do? Come, come, come girl. Come an sit down. Queenie, child, me mind did tell me you mother would send you up today."

Cousin Kamay accepted their arrival as a matter of course.

"Constance, put some food in the bowl for Cousin Liza. Go in the kitchen an see what you get to eat, Queen. It have food dey. Help youself to what you want. How you mother?"

"She well tanks."

"Well tanks *who?*"

"She well tanks, Cousin Kamay."

Cousin Kamay watched her. "Hm! You gettin big! These children nowadays you have to keep a eye on them yes. Go an see what you get to eat!"

The journey was over. In two days' time, after being about her mother's business, eleven-year-old Queen would leave again with Cousin Liza or whoever else happened to be making the trip to St David's. The one thing that remained to haunt her was the knowledge that the return trip would have to be made in darkness, when the sun was down, and when those who had to walk always made their journeys.

Rainer Maria Rilke
A WALK

Translated by Roger Gilbert

Already my gaze is on the hill, that sunny one
Far ahead on the path I've just begun.
So held are we by what we cannot hold,
It looks full of vision, from a distance.

And even if we never get there, it changes us
Into what we'll hardly guess we are.
A signal moves, mirroring our own.
Yet we only feel the headwind.

Gary Snyder
A WALK

Sunday the only day we don't work:
Mules farting around the meadow,
       Murphy fishing,
The tent flaps in the warm
Early sun: I've eaten breakfast and I'll
       take a walk
To Benson Lake. Packed a lunch,
Goodbye. Hopping on creekbed boulders
Up the rock throat three miles
       Piute Creek—
In steep gorge glacier-slick rattlesnake country
Jump, land by a pool, trout skitter,
The clear sky. Deer tracks.
Bad place by a falls, boulders big as houses,
Lunch tied to belt,
I stemmed up a crack and almost fell
But rolled out safe on a ledge
       and ambled on.
Quail chicks freeze underfoot, color of stone
Then run cheep! away, hen quail fussing.
Craggy west end of Benson Lake—after edging
Past dark creek pools on a long white slope—
Lookt down in the ice-black lake
       lined with cliff
From far above: deep shimmering trout.
A lone duck in a gunsightpass
       steep side hill
Through slide-aspen and talus, to the east end,

Down to grass, wading a wide smooth stream
Into camp. At last.
  By the rusty three-year-
Ago left-behind cookstove
Of the old trail crew,
Stoppt and swam and ate my lunch.

Edward Abbey
WALKING

Whenever possible I avoid the practice myself. If God had meant us to walk, he would have kept us down on all fours, with well-padded paws. He would have constructed our planet on the model of the simple cube, so that the notion of circularity and consequently the wheel might never have arisen. He surely would not have made mountains.

There is something unnatural about walking. Especially walking uphill, which always seems to me not only unnatural but so *unnecessary*. That iron tug of gravitation should be all the reminder we need that in walking uphill we are violating a basic law of nature. Yet we persist in doing it. No one can explain why. George H. Leigh-Mallory's asinine rationale for climbing a mountain—"because it's there"—could easily be refuted with a few well-placed hydrogen bombs. But our common sense continues to lag far behind the available technology.

My own first Group Outing was with the United States Infantry. The experience made a bad impression on my psyche—a blister on my soul that has never healed completely. Of course, we were outfitted with the very best hiking equipment the army could provide: heavy-gauge steel helmet; gas mask; knee-length wool overcoat; fully loaded ammunition belt around the waist, resting on the kidneys; full field pack including a shovel ("entrenching tool"), a rugged canvas tarpaulin ("shelter half") and a pair of wool blankets for bivouac; steel canteen filled with briny water (our group leader insisted on dumping salt tablets into each member's canteen at the beginning of the hike); and such obvious essentials as combat boots, bayonet, and the M-1 rifle. Since resigning from the infantry, some time ago, I have not participated in any group outings.

However, some of us do walk best under duress. Or only under duress. Certainly my own most memorable hikes can be classified as Shortcuts that Backfired. For example, showing my wife the easy way to drive down from

Deadhorse Point to Moab, via Pucker Pass, I took a wrong turn in the twilight, got lost in a maze of jeep trails, ran out of gas. We walked about twenty miles that night, through the rain, she in tennis shoes and me in cowboy boots. Better than waiting for the heat of the day. Or take the time I tried to force a Hertz rented car up Elephant Hill on the Needles Jeep Trail—another long, impromptu walk. Or one night on the eastern outskirts of Albuquerque, New Mexico, when a bunch of student drunks decided to climb the Sandia Mountains by moonlight. About twelve started; two of us made it, arriving at the crest sixteen hours later, famished, disillusioned, lacerated, and exhausted. But it sure cured the hangover.

There are some good things to say about walking. Not many, but some. Walking takes longer, for example, than any other known form of locomotion except crawling. Thus is stretches time and prolongs life. Life is already too short to waste on speed. I have a friend who's always in a hurry; he never gets anywhere. Walking makes the world much bigger and therefore more interesting. You have time to observe the details. The utopian technologists foresee a future for us in which distance is annihilated and anyone can transport himself anywhere, instantly. Big deal, Buckminster. To be everywhere at once is to be nowhere forever, if you ask me. That's God's job, not ours; that's what we pay Him for. Her for.

The longest journey begins with a single step, not with a turn of the ignition key. That's the best thing about walking, the journey itself. It doesn't much matter whether you get where you're going or not. You'll get there anyway. Every good hike brings you eventually back home. Right where you started.

Which reminds me of circles. Which reminds me of wheels. Which reminds me my old truck needs another front-end job. Any good mechanics out there wandering through the smog?

Linda Hogan
WALKING

It began in dark and underground weather, a slow hunger moving toward light. It grew in a dry gulley beside the road where I live, a place where entire hillsides are sometimes yellow, windblown tides of sunflower plants. But this plant was different. It was alone and larger than the countless others that had established their lives farther up the hill. This one was a traveler, a settler, and like a dream beginning in conflict, it grew where the land had been disturbed.

I saw it first in early summer. It was a green and sleeping bud, raising itself toward the sun. Ants worked around the unopened bloom, gathering aphids and sap. A few days later, it was a tender young flower, soft and new, with a pale green center and a troop of silver-gray insects climbing up and down the stalk. Over the summer this sunflower grew into a plant of incredible beauty, turning its face daily toward the sun in the most subtle of ways, the black center of it dark and alive with a deep blue light, as if flint had sparked an elemental fire there, in community with rain, mineral, mountain air, and sand.

As summer changed from green to yellow there were new visitors daily, the lace-winged insects, the bees whose legs were fat with pollen, and grasshoppers with their clattering wings and desperate hunger. There were other lives I missed, those too small or hidden to see. It was as if this plant with its host of lives was a society, one in which moment by moment, depending on light and moisture, there was great and diverse change.

There were changes in the next larger world around the plant as well. One day I rounded a bend in the road to find the disturbing sight of a dead horse, black and still against a hillside, eyes rolled back. Another day I was nearly lifted by a wind and sandstorm so fierce and hot that I had to wait for it to pass before I could return home, On this day the faded dry petals of the sunflower were swept across the land. That was when the birds arrived to carry the new seeds to another future.

In this one plant, in one summer season, a drama of need and survival took place. Hungers were filled. Insects coupled. There was escape, exhaustion, and death. Lives touched down a moment and were gone.

I was an outsider. I only watched. I never learned the sunflower's golden language or the tongues of its citizens. I had a small understanding, nothing more than a shallow observation of the flower, insects, and birds. But they knew what to do, how to live. An old voice from somewhere, gene or cell, told the plant how to evade the pull of gravity and find its way upward, how to open. It was instinct, intuition, necessity. A certain knowing directed the seed-bearing birds on paths to ancestral homelands they had never seen. They believed it. They followed.

There are other summons and calls, some even more mysterious than those commandments to birds or those survival journeys of insects. In bamboo plants, for instance, with their thin green canopy of light and golden stalks that creak in the wind. Once a century, all of a certain kind of bamboo flower on the same day. Neither the plants' location, in Malaysia or in a greenhouse in Minnesota, nor their age or size make a difference. They flower. Some current of an inner language passes among them, through space and separation, in ways we cannot explain in our language. They are all, somehow, one plant, each with a share of communal knowledge.

John Hay, in *The Immortal Wilderness,* has written: "There are occasions when you can hear the mysterious language of the Earth, in water, or coming through the trees, emanating from the mosses, seeping through the undercurrents of the soil, but you have to be willing to wait and receive."

Sometimes I hear it talking. The light of the sunflower was one language, but there are others more audible. Once, in the redwood forest, I heard a beat, something like a drum or heart coming from the ground and trees and wind. That underground current stirred a kind of knowing inside me, a kinship and longing, a dream barely remembered that disappeared back to the body. Another time, there was the booming voice of an ocean storm thundering from far out at sea, telling about what lived in the distance, about the tough water that would arrive, wave after wave revealing the disturbance at center.

Tonight I walk. I am watching the sky. I think of the people who came before me and how they knew the placement of stars in the, sky, watched the moving sun long and hard enough to witness how a certain angle of light touched a stone only once a year. Without written records, they knew the gods of every night, the small, fine details of the world around them and of immensity above them.

Walking, I can almost hear the redwoods beating. And the oceans are above me here, rolling clouds, heavy and dark, considering snow. On the dry, red road, I pass the place of the sunflower, that dark and secret location where creation took place. I wonder if it will return this summer, if it will multiply and move up to the other stand of flowers in a territorial struggle.

It's winter and there is smoke from the fires. The square, lighted windows of houses are fogging over. It is a world of elemental attention, of all things working together, listening to what speaks in the blood. Whichever road I follow, I walk in the land of many gods, and they love and eat one another. Walking, I am listening to a deeper way. Suddenly all my ancestors are behind me. Be still, they say. Watch and listen. You are the result of the love of thousands.

Thomas Traherne
WALKING

To walk abroad is, not with eyes,
But thoughts, the fields to see and prize;
 Else may the silent feet,
  Like logs of wood,
Move up and down, and see no good
 Nor joy nor glory meet.

Ev'n carts and wheels their place do change,
But cannot see, though very strange
 The glory that is by;
  Dead puppets may
Move in the bright and glorious day,
 Yet not behold the sky.

And are not men than they more blind,
Who having eyes yet never find
 The bliss in which they move;
  Like statues dead
They up and down are carried
 Yet never see nor love.

To walk is by a thought to go;
To move in spirit to and fro;
 To mind the good we see;
  To taste the sweet;
Observing all the things we meet
 How choice and rich they be.

To note the beauty of the day,
And golden fields of corn survey;
　　Admire each pretty flow'r
　　　With its sweet smell;
To praise their Maker, and to tell
　　The marks of his great pow'r.

To fly abroad like active bees,
Among the hedges and the trees,
　　To cull the dew that lies
　　　On ev'ry blade,
From ev'ry blossom; till we lade
　　Our minds, as they their thighs.

Observe those rich and glorious things,
The rivers, meadows, woods, and springs,
　　The fructifying sun;
　　　To note from far
The rising of each twinkling star
　　For us his race to run.

A little child these well perceives,
Who, tumbling in green grass and leaves,
　　May rich as kings be thought,
　　　But there's a sight
Which perfect manhood may delight,
　　To which we shall be brought.

While in those pleasant paths we talk,
'Tis that tow'rds which at last we walk;
　　For we may by degrees
　　　Wisely proceed
Pleasures of love and praise to heed,
　　From viewing herbs and trees.

Pablo Neruda
WALKING AROUND

Translated by Robert Bly

It so happens I am sick of being a man.
And it happens that I walk into tailorshops and movie houses
dried up, waterproof, like a swan made of felt
steering my way in a water of wombs and ashes.

The smell of barbershops makes me break into hoarse sobs.
The only thing I want is to lie still like stones or wool.
The only thing I want is to see no more stores, no gardens,
no more goods, no spectacles, no elevators.

It so happens I am sick of my feet and my nails
and my hair and my shadow.
It so happens I am sick of being a man.

Still it would be marvelous
to terrify a law clerk with a cut lily,
or kill a nun with a blow on the ear.
It would be great
to go through the streets with a green knife
letting out yells until I died of the cold.

I don't want to go on being a root in the dark,
insecure, stretched out, shivering with sleep,
going on down, into the moist guts of the earth,
taking in and thinking, eating every day.

I don't want so much misery.
I don't want to go on as a root and a tomb,
alone under the ground, a warehouse with corpses,
half frozen, dying of grief.

That's why Monday, when it sees me coming
with my convict face, blazes up like gasoline,
and it howls on its way like a wounded wheel,
and leaves tracks full of warm blood leading toward the night.

And it pushes me into certain corners, into some moist houses,
into hospitals where the bones fly out the window,
into shoeshops that smell like vinegar,
and certain streets hideous as cracks in the skin.

There are sulphur-colored birds, and hideous intestines
hanging over the doors of houses that I hate,
and there are false teeth forgotten in a coffeepot,
there are mirrors
that ought to have wept from shame and terror,
there are umbrellas everywhere, and venoms, and umbilical cords.

I stroll along serenely, with my eyes, my shoes,
my rage, forgetting everything,
I walk by, going through office buildings and orthopedic shops,
and courtyards with washing hanging from the line:
underwear, towels and shirts from which slow
dirty tears are falling.

Audre Lorde
WALKING OUR BOUNDARIES

This first bright day has broken
the back of winter.
We rise from war
to walk across the earth
around our house
both stunned that sun can shine so brightly
after all our pain
Cautiously we inspect our joint holding.
A part of last year's garden still stands
bracken
one tough missed okra pod clings to the vine
a parody of fruit cold-hard and swollen
underfoot
one rotting shingle
is becoming loam.

I take your hand beside the compost heap
glad to be alive and still
with you
we talk of ordinary articles
with relief
while we peer upward
each half-afraid
there will be no tight buds started
on our ancient apple tree
so badly damaged by last winter's storm
knowing
it does not pay to cherish symbols

when the substance
lies so close at hand
waiting to be held
your hand
falls off the apple bark
like casual fire
along my back
my shoulders are dead leaves
waiting to be burned
to life.

The sun is watery warm
our voices
seem too loud for this small yard
too tentative for women
so in love
the siding has come loose in spots
our footsteps hold this place
together
as our place
our joint decisions make the possible
whole.
I do not know when
we shall laugh again
but next week
we will spade up another plot
for this spring's seeding.

William Wordsworth
WHEN, TO THE ATTRACTIONS OF
THE BUSY WORLD

When, to the attractions of the busy world,
Preferring studious leisure, I had chosen
A habitation in this peaceful Vale,
Sharp season followed of continual storm
In deepest winter; and, from week to week,
Pathway, and lane, and public road, were clogged
With frequent showers of snow. Upon a hill
At a short distance from my cottage, stands
A stately Fir-grove, whither I was wont
To hasten, for I found, beneath the roof
Of that perennial shade, a cloistral place
Of refuge, with an unincumbered floor.
Here, in safe covert, on the shallow snow,
And, sometimes, on a speck of visible earth,
The redbreast near me hopped; nor was I loth
To sympathise with vulgar coppice birds
That, for protection from the nipping blast,
Hither repaired.—A single beech-tree grew
Within this grove of firs! and, on the fork
Of that one beech, appeared a thrush's nest;
A last year's nest, conspicuously built
At such small elevation from the ground
As gave sure sign that they, who in that house
Of nature and of love had made their home
Amid the fir-trees, all the summer long
Dwelt in a tranquil spot. And oftentimes,
A few sheep, stragglers from some mountain-flock,

Would watch my motions with suspicious stare,
From the remotest outskirts of the grove,—
Some nook where they had made their final stand,
Huddling together from two fears—the fear
Of me and of the storm. Full many an hour
Here did I lose. But in this grove the trees
Had been so thickly planted, and had thriven
In such perplexed and intricate array;
That vainly did I seek, beneath their stems
A length of open space, where to and fro
My feet might move without concern or care;
And, baffled thus, though earth from day to day
Was fettered, and the air by storm disturbed,
I ceased the shelter to frequent,—and prized,
Less than I wished to prize, that calm recess.

   The snows dissolved, and genial Spring returned
To clothe the fields with verdure. Other haunts
Meanwhile were mine; till, one bright April day,
By chance retiring from the glare of noon
To this forsaken covert, there I found
A hoary pathway traced between the trees,
And winding on with such an easy line
Along a natural opening, that I stood
Much wondering how I could have sought in vain
For what was now so obvious. To abide,
For an allotted interval of ease,
Under my cottage-roof, had gladly come
From the wild sea a cherished Visitant;
And with the sight of this same path—begun,
Begun and ended, in the shady grove,
Pleasant conviction flashed upon my mind
That, to this opportune recess allured,
He had surveyed it with a finer eye,
A heart more wakeful; and had worn the track
By pacing here, unwearied and alone,

In that habitual restlessness of foot
That haunts the Sailor measuring o'er and o'er
His short domain upon the vessel's deck,
While she pursues her course through the dreary sea.
   When thou hadst quitted Esthwaite's pleasant shore,
And taken thy first leave of those green hills
And rocks that were the play-ground of thy youth,
Year followed year, my Brother! and we two,
Conversing not, knew little in what mould
Each other's mind was fashioned; and at length,
When once again we met in Grasmere Vale,
Between us there was little other bond
Than common feelings of fraternal love.
But thou, a Schoolboy, to the sea hadst carried
Undying recollections! Nature there
Was with thee; she, who loved us both, she still
Was with thee; and even so didst thou become
A 'silent' Poet; from the solitude
Of the vast sea didst bring a watchful heart
Still couchant, an inevitable ear,
And an eye practised like a blind man's touch.
—Back to the joyless Ocean thou art gone;
Nor from this vestige of thy musing hours
Could I withhold thy honoured name,—and now
I love the fir-grove with a perfect love.
Thither do I withdraw when cloudless suns
Shine hot, or wind blows troublesome and strong;
And there I sit at evening, when the steep
Of Silver-how, and Grasmere's peaceful lake,
And one green island, gleam between the stems
Of the dark firs, a visionary scene!
And, while I gaze upon the spectacle
Of clouded splendour, on this dream-like sight
Of solemn loveliness, I think on thee,
My Brother, and on all which thou hast lost.

Nor seldom, if I rightly guess, while Thou,
Muttering the verses which I muttered first
Among the mountains, through the midnight watch
Art pacing thoughtfully the vessel's deck
In some far region, here, while o'er my head,
At every impulse of the moving breeze,
The fir-grove murmurs with a sea-like sound,
Alone I tread this path;—for aught I know,
Timing my steps to thine; and, with a store
Of undistinguishable sympathies,
Mingling most earnest wishes for the day
When we, and others whom we love, shall meet
A second time, in Grasmere's happy Vale.

D. H. Lawrence
THE WILD COMMON

The quick sparks on the gorse bushes are leaping,
Little jets of sunlight-texture imitating flame;
Above them, exultant, the pee-wits are sweeping:
They are lords of the desolate wastes of sadness their screamings proclaim.

Rabbits, handfuls of brown earth, lie
Low-rounded on the mournful grass they have bitten down to the quick.
Are they asleep?—Are they alive?—Now see, when I
Move my arms the hill bursts and heaves under their spurting kick.

The common flaunts bravely; but below, from the rushes
Crowds of glittering king-cups surge to challenge the blossoming bushes;
There the lazy streamlet pushes
Its curious course mildly; here it wakes again, leaps, laughs, and gushes.

Into a deep pond, an old sheep-dip,
Dark, overgrown with willows, cool, with the brook ebbing through so slow,
Naked on the steep, soft lip
Of the bank I stand watching my own white shadow quivering to and fro.

What if the gorse flowers shrivelled and kissing were lost?
Without the pulsing waters, where were the marigolds and the songs of the
    brook?
If my veins and my breasts with love embossed
Withered, my insolent soul would be gone like flowers that the hot wind took.

So my soul like a passionate woman turns,
Filled with remorseful terror to the man she scorned, and her love

For myself in my own eyes' laughter burns,
Runs ecstatic over the pliant folds rippling down to my belly from the breast-
   lights above.

Over my sunlit skin the warm, clinging air,
Rich with the songs of seven larks singing at once, goes kissing me glad.
And the soul of the wind and my blood compare
Their wandering happiness, and the wind, wasted in liberty, drifts on and is
   sad.

Oh but the water loves me and folds me,
Plays with me, sways me, lifts me and sinks me as though it were living blood,
Blood of a heaving woman who holds me,
Owning my supple body a rare glad thing, supremely good.

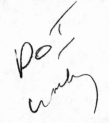

Henry David Thoreau
A WINTER WALK

The wind has gently murmured through the blinds, or puffed with feathery softness against the windows, and occasionally sighed like a summer zephyr lifting the leaves along, the livelong night. The meadow mouse has slept in his snug gallery in the sod, the owl has sat in a hollow tree in the depth of the swamp, the rabbit, the squirrel, and the fox have all been housed. The watchdog has lain quiet on the hearth, and the cattle have stood silent in their stalls. The earth itself has slept, as it were its first, not its last sleep, save when some street sign or woodhouse door has faintly creaked upon its hinge, cheering forlorn nature at her midnight work—the only sound awake 'twixt Venus and Mars—advertising us of a remote inward warmth, a divine cheer and fellowship, where gods are met together, but where it is very bleak for men to stand. But while the earth has slumbered, all the air has been alive with feathery flakes descending, as if some northern Ceres reigned, showering her silvery grain over all the fields.

We sleep, and at length awake to the still reality of a winter morning. The snow lies warm as cotton or down upon the window sill; the broadened sash and frosted panes admit a dim and private light, which enhances the snug cheer within. The stillness of the morning is impressive. The floor creaks under our feet as we move toward the window to look abroad through some clear space over the fields. We see the roofs stand under their snow burden. From the eaves and fences hang stalactites of snow, and in the yard stand stalagmites covering some concealed core. The trees and shrubs rear white arms to the sky on every side; and where were walls and fences, we see fantastic forms stretching in frolic gambols across the dusky landscape, as if Nature had strewn her fresh designs over the fields by night as models for man's art.

Silently we unlatch the door, letting the drift fall in, and step abroad to face the cutting air. Already the stars have lost some of their sparkle, and a dull, leaden mist skirts the horizon. A lurid brazen light in the east proclaims the

approach of day, while the western landscape is dim and spectral still, and
clothed in a somber Tartarean light, like the shadowy realms. They are
Infernal sounds only that you hear—the crowing of cocks, the barking of dogs,
the chopping of wood, the lowing of kine, all seem to come from Pluto's barn-
yard and beyond the Styx—not for any melancholy they suggest, but their twilight bustle is too solemn and mysterious for earth. The recent tracks of the fox
or otter, in the yard, remind us that each hour of the night is crowded with
events, and the primeval nature is still working and making tracks in the snow.
Opening the gate, we tread briskly along the lone country road, crunching the
dry and crisped snow under our feet, or aroused by the sharp, clear creak of
the wood sled, just starting for the distant market, from the early farmer's door,
where it has lain the summer long, dreaming amid the chips and stubble;
while far through the drifts and powdered windows we see the farmer's early
candle, like a paled star, emitting a lonely beam, as if some severe virtue were
at its matins there. And one by one the smokes begin to ascend from the chimneys amid the trees and snows.

    The sluggish smoke curls up from some deep dell,
    The stiffened air exploring in the dawn,
    And making slow acquaintance with the day
    Delaying now upon its heavenward course,
    In wreathèd loiterings dallying with itself,
    With as uncertain purpose and slow deed
    As its half-awakened master by the hearth,
    Whose mind still slumbering and sluggish thoughts
    Have not yet swept into the onward current
    Of the new day—and now it streams afar,
    The while the chopper goes with step direct,
    And mind intent to swing the early axe.
        First in the dusky dawn he sends abroad
    His early scout, his emissary, smoke,
    The earliest, latest pilgrim from the roof,
    To feel the frosty air, inform the day;
    And while he crouches still beside the hearth,
    Nor musters courage to unbar the door,

It has gone down the glen with the light wind,
And o'er the plain unfurled its venturous wreath,
Draped the treetops, loitered upon the hill,
And warmed the pinions of the early bird;
And now, perchance, high in the crispy air,
Has caught sight of the day o'er the earth's edge,
And greets its master's eye at his low door,
As some refulgent cloud in the upper sky.

We hear the sound of woodchopping at the farmers' doors, far over the frozen earth, the baying of the house dog, and the distant clarion of the cock —though the thin and frosty air conveys only the finer particles of sound to our ears, with short and sweet vibrations, as the waves subside soonest on the purest and lightest liquids, in which gross substances sink to the bottom. They come clear and bell-like, and from a greater distance in the horizon, as if there were fewer impediments than in summer to make them faint and ragged. The ground is sonorous, like seasoned wood, and even the ordinary rural sounds are melodious, and the jingling of the ice on the trees is sweet and liquid. There is the least possible moisture in the atmosphere, all being dried up or congealed, and it is of such extreme tenuity and elasticity that it becomes a source of delight. The withdrawn and tense sky seems groined like the aisles of a cathedral, and the polished air sparkles as if there were crystals of ice floating in it. As they who have resided in Greenland tell us that when it freezes "the sea smokes like burning turf-land, and a fog or mist arises, called frost-smoke," which "cutting smoke frequently raises blisters on the face and hands, and is very pernicious to the health." But this pure, stinging cold is an elixir to the lungs, and not so much a frozen mist as a crystallized midsummer haze, refined and purified by cold.

The sun at length rises through the distant woods, as if with the faint clashing, swinging sound of cymbals, melting the air with his beams, and with such rapid steps the morning travels, that already his rays are gilding the distant western mountains. Meanwhile we step hastily along through the powdery snow, warmed by an inward heat, enjoying an Indian summer still, in the increased glow of thought and feeling. Probably if our lives were more conformed to nature, we should not need to defend ourselves against her heats and colds, but find her our constant nurse and friend, as do plants and quadrupeds. If our bodies were fed with pure and simple elements, and not with a stimulating and heating diet, they would afford no more pasture for cold than a leafless twig, but thrive like the trees, which find even winter genial to their expansion.

The wonderful purity of nature at this season is a most pleasing fact. Every decayed stump and moss-grown stone and rail, and the dead leaves of autumn, are concealed by a clean napkin of snow. In the bare fields and tinkling woods, see what virtue survives. In the coldest and bleakest places, the warmest charities still maintain a foothold. A cold and searching wind drives away all contagion, and nothing can withstand it but what has a virtue in it, and accordingly, whatever we meet with in cold and bleak places, as the tops of mountains, we respect for a sort of sturdy innocence, a Puritan toughness. All things beside seem to be called in for shelter, and what stays out must be part of the original frame of the universe, and of such valor as God himself. It is invigorating to breathe the cleansed air. Its greater fineness and purity are visible to the eye, and we would fain stay out long and late, that the gales may sigh through us, too, as through the leafless trees, and fit us for the winter—as if we hoped so to borrow some pure and steadfast virtue, which will stead us in all seasons.

There is a slumbering subterranean fire in nature which never goes out, and which no cold can chill. It finally melts the great snow, and in January or July is only buried under a thicker or thinner covering. In the coldest day it flows somewhere, and the snow melts around every tree. This field of winter rye, which sprouted late in the fall, and now speedily dissolves the snow, is where the fire is very thinly covered. We feel warmed by it. In the winter, warmth stands for all virtue, and we resort in thought to a trickling rill, with its bare stones shining in the sun, and to warm springs in the woods, with as much eagerness as rabbits and robins. The steam which rises from swamps and pools is as dear and domestic as that of our own kettle. What fire could ever equal the sunshine of a winter's day, when the meadow mice come out by the wall-sides, and the chickadee lisps in the defiles of the wood? The warmth comes directly from the sun, and is not radiated from the earth, as in summer; and when we feel his beams on our backs as we are treading some snowy dell, we are grateful as for a special kindness, and bless the sun which has followed us into that by-place.

This subterranean fire has its altar in each man's breast; for in the coldest day, and on the bleakest hill, the traveler cherishes a warmer fire within the folds of his cloak than is kindled on any hearth. A healthy man, indeed, is the complement of the seasons, and in winter, summer is in his heart. There is the south. Thither have all birds and insects migrated, and around the warm springs in his breast are gathered the robin and the lark.

At length, having reached the edge of the woods, and shut out the gadding town, we enter within their covert as we go under the roof of a cottage, and cross its threshold; all ceiled and banked up with snow. They are glad and warm still, and as genial and cheery in winter as in summer. As we stand in the midst of the pines in the flickering and checkered light which straggles but little way into their maze, we wonder if the towns have ever heard their simple story. It seems to us that no traveler has ever explored them, and notwithstanding the wonders which science is elsewhere revealing every day, who would not like to hear their annals? Our humble villages in the plain are their contribution. We borrow from the forest the boards which shelter and the sticks which warm us. How important is their evergreen to the winter, that portion of the summer which does not fade, the permanent year, the unwithered grass! Thus simply, and with little expense of altitude, is the surface of the earth diversified. What would human life be without forests, those natural cities? From the tops of mountains they appear like smooth-shaven lawns, yet whither shall we walk but in this taller grass?

In this glade covered with bushes of a year's growth, see how the silvery dust lies on every seared leaf and twig, deposited in such infinite and luxurious forms as by their very variety atone for the absence of color. Observe the tiny tracks of mice around every stem, and the triangular tracks of the rabbit. A pure elastic heaven hangs over all, as if the impurities of the summer sky, refined and shrunk by the chaste winter's cold, had been winnowed from the heavens upon the earth.

Nature confounds her summer distinctions at this season. The heavens seem to be nearer the earth. The elements are less reserved and distinct. Water turns to ice, rain to snow. The day is but a Scandinavian night. The winter is an arctic summer.

How much more living is the life that is in nature, the furred life which still survives the stinging nights, and, from amidst fields and woods covered with frost and snow, sees the sun rise!

"The foodless wilds
Pour forth their brown inhabitants."

The gray squirrel and rabbit are brisk and playful in the remote glens, even on the morning of the cold Friday. Here is our Lapland and Labrador, and for our Esquimaux and Knistenaux, Dog-ribbed Indians, Novazemblaites, and Spitzbergeners, are there not the ice-cutter and woodchopper, the fox, muskrat, and mink?

Still, in the midst of the arctic day, we may trace the summer to its retreats, and sympathize with some contemporary life. Stretched over the brooks, in the midst of the frost-bound meadows, we may observe the submarine cottages of the caddis-worms, the larvae of the Plicipennes; their small cylindrical cases built around themselves, composed of flags, sticks, grass, and withered leaves, shells, and pebbles, in form and color like the wrecks which strew the bottom,—now drifting along over the pebbly bottom, now whirling in tiny eddies and dashing down steep falls, or sweeping rapidly along with the current, or else swaying to and fro at the end of some grass-blade or root. Anon they will leave their sunken habitations, and, crawling up the stems of plants, or to the surface, like gnats, as perfect insects henceforth, flutter over the surface of the water, or sacrifice their short lives in the flame of our candles at evening. Down yonder little glen the shrubs are drooping under their burden, and the red alderberries contrast with the white ground. Here are the marks of a myriad feet which have already been abroad. The sun rises as proudly over such a glen as over the valley of the Seine or the Tiber, and it seems the residence of a pure and self-subsistent valor, such as they never witnessed—which never knew defeat nor fear. Here reign the simplicity and purity of a primitive age, and a health and hope far remote from towns and cities. Standing quite alone, far in the forest, while the wind is shaking down snow from the trees, and leaving the only human tracks behind us, we find our reflections of a richer variety than the life of cities. The chickadee and nuthatch are more inspiring society than statesmen and philosophers, and we shall return to these last as to more vulgar companions. In this lonely glen, with its brook draining the slopes, its creased ice and crystals of all hues, where the spruces and hemlocks stand up on either side, and the rush and sere wild oats in the rivulet itself, our lives are more serene and worthy to contemplate.

As the day advances, the heat of the sun is reflected by the hillsides, and we hear a faint but sweet music, where flows the rill released from its fetters, and the icicles are melting on the trees; and the nuthatch and partridge are heard and seen. The south wind melts the snow at noon, and the bare ground appears with its withered grass and leaves, and we are invigorated by the perfume which exhales from it, as by the scent of strong meats.

Let us go into this deserted woodman's hut, and see how he has passed the long winter nights and the short and stormy days. For here man has lived under this south hillside, and it seems a civilized and public spot. We have such associations as when the traveler stands by the ruins of Palmyra or Hecatompolis. Singing birds and flowers perchance have begun to appear here, for flowers as well as weeds follow in the footsteps of man. These hemlocks whispered over his head, these hickory logs were his fuel, and these pitch pine roots kindled his fire; yonder fuming rill in the hollow, whose thin and airy vapor still ascends as busily as ever, though he is far off now, was his well. These hemlock boughs, and the straw upon this raised platform, were his bed, and this broken dish held his drink. But he has not been here this season, for the phoebes built their nest upon this shelf last summer. I find some embers left as if he had but just gone out, where he baked his pot of beans; and while at evening he smoked his pipe, whose stemless bowl lies in the ashes, chatted with his only companion, if perchance he had any, about the depth of the snow on the morrow, already falling fast and thick without, or disputed whether the last sound was the screech of an owl, or the creak of a bough, or imagination only; and through his broad chimney-throat, in the late winter evening, ere he stretched himself upon the straw, he looked up to learn the progress of the storm, and, seeing the bright stars of Cassiopeia's Chair shining brightly down upon him, fell contentedly asleep.

See how many traces from which we may learn the chopper's history! From this stamp we may guess the sharpness of his axe, and from the slope of the stroke, on which side he stood, and whether he cut down the tree without going round it or changing hands; and, from the flexure of the splinters, we may know which way it fell. This one chip contains inscribed on it the whole history of the woodchopper and of the world. On this scrap of paper, which held his sugar or salt, perchance, or was the wadding of his gun, sitting on a log in the forest, with what interest we read the tattle of cities, of those larger huts, empty and to let, like this, in High Streets and Broadways. The eaves are dripping on the south side of this simple roof, while the titmouse lisps in the pine and the genial warmth of the sun around the door is somewhat kind and human.

After two seasons, this rude dwelling does not deform the scene. Already the birds resort to it, to build their nests, and you may track to its door the feet of many quadrupeds. Thus, for a long time, nature overlooks the encroachment and profanity of man. The wood still cheerfully and unsuspiciously echoes the strokes of the axe that fells it, and while they are few and seldom, they enhance its wildness, and all the elements strive to naturalize the sound.

Now our path begins to ascend gradually to the top of this high hill, from whose precipitous south side we can look over the broad country of forest and field and river, to the distant snowy mountains. See yonder thin column of smoke curling up through the woods from some invisible farmhouse, the standard raised over some rural homestead. There must be a warmer and more genial spot there below, as where we detect the vapor from a spring forming a cloud above the trees. What fine relations are established between the traveler who discovers this airy column from some eminence in the forest and him who sits below! Up goes the smoke as silently and naturally as the vapor exhales from the leaves, and as busy disposing itself in wreaths as the housewife on the hearth below. It is a hieroglyphic of man's life, and suggests more intimate and important things than the boiling of a pot. Where its fine column rises above the forest, like an ensign, some human life has planted itself—and such is the beginning of Rome, the establishment of the arts, and the foundation of empires, whether on the prairies of America or the steppes of Asia.

And now we descend again, to the brink of this woodland lake, which lies in a hollow of the hills, as if it were their expressed juice, and that of the leaves which are annually steeped in it. Without outlet or inlet to the eye, it has still its history, in the lapse of its waves, in the rounded pebbles on its shore, and in the pines which grow down to its brink. It has not been idle, though sedentary, but, like Abu Musa, teaches that "sitting still at home is the heavenly way; the going out is the way of the world." Yet in its evaporation it travels as far as any.

In summer it is the earth's liquid eye, a mirror in the breast of nature. The sins of the wood are washed out in it. See how the woods form an amphitheater about it, and it is an arena for all the genialness of nature. All trees direct the traveler to its brink, all paths seek it out, birds fly to it, quadrupeds flee to it, and the very ground inclines toward it. It is nature's saloon, where she has sat down to her toilet. Consider her silent economy and tidiness; how the sun comes with his evaporation to sweep the dust from its surface each morning, and a fresh surface is constantly welling up; and annually, after whatever impurities have accumulated herein, its liquid transparency appears again in the spring. In summer a hushed music seems to sweep across its surface. But now a plain sheet of snow conceals it from our eyes, except where the wind has swept the ice bare, and the sere leaves are gliding from side to side, tacking and veering on their tiny voyages. Here is one just keeled up against a pebble on shore, a dry beech leaf, rocking still, as if it would start again. A skillful engineer, methinks, might project its course since it fell from the parent stem. Here are all the elements for such a calculation. Its present position, the direction of the wind, the level of the pond, and how much more is given. In its scarred edges and veins is its log rolled up.

We fancy ourselves in the interior of a larger house. The surface of the pond is our deal table or sanded floor, and the woods rise abruptly from its edge, like the walls of a cottage. The lines set to catch pickerel through the ice look like a larger culinary preparation, and the men stand about on the white ground like pieces of forest furniture. The actions of these men, at the distance of half a mile over the ice and snow, impress us as when we read the exploits of Alexander in history. They seem not unworthy of the scenery, and as momentous as the conquest of kingdoms.

Again we have wandered through the arches of the wood, until from its skirts we hear the distant booming of ice from yonder bay of the river, as if it were moved by some other and subtler tide than oceans know. To me it has a strange sound of home, thrilling as the voice of one's distant and noble kindred. A mild summer sun shines over forest and lake, and though there is but one green leaf for many rocks, yet nature enjoys a serene health. Every sound is fraught with the same mysterious assurance of health, as well now the creaking of the boughs in January, as the soft sough of the wind in July.

When Winter fringes every bough
  With his fantastic wreath,
And puts the seal of silence now
  Upon the leaves beneath;

When every stream in its penthouse
  Goes gurgling on its way,
And in his gallery the mouse
  Nibbleth the meadow hay;

Methinks the summer still is nigh,
  And lurketh underneath,
As that same meadow mouse doth lie
  Snug in the last year's heath.

And if perchance the chickadee
  Lisp a faint note anon,
The snow in summer's canopy,
  Which she herself put on.

Fair blossoms deck the cheerful trees,
  And dazzling fruits depend,
The north wind sighs a summer breeze,
  The nipping frosts to fend,

Bringing glad tidings unto me,
  The while I stand all ear,
Of a serene eternity,
  Which need not winter fear.

Out on the silent pond straightway
  The restless ice doth crack,
And pond sprites merry gambols play
  Amid the deafening rack.

Eager I hasten to the vale,
  As if I heard brave news,
How nature held high festival,
  Which it were hard to lose.

I gambol with my neighbor ice,
  And sympathizing quake,
As each new crack darts in a trice
  Across the gladsome lake.

One with the cricket in the ground,
  And faggot on the hearth,
Resounds the rare domestic sound
  Along the forest path.

Before night we will take a journey on skates along the course of this meandering river, as full of novelty to one who sits by the cottage fire all the winter's
day, as if it were over the polar ice, with Captain Parry or Franklin; following
the winding of the stream, now flowing amid hills, now spreading out into fair
meadows, and forming a myriad coves and bays where the pine and hemlock
overarch. The river flows in the rear of the towns, and we see all things from a
new and wilder side. The fields and gardens come down. to it with a frankness, and freedom from pretension, which they do not wear on the highway. It
is the outside and edge of the earth. Our eyes are not offended by violent con-
trasts. The last rail of the farmer's fence is some swaying willow boughs,
which still preserves its freshness, and here at length all fences stop, and we no
longer cross any road. We may go far up within the country now by the most
retired and level road, never climbing a hill, but by broad levels ascending to
the upland meadows. It is a beautiful illustration of the law of obedience, the
flow of a river; the path for a sick man, a highway down which an acorn cup
may float secure with its freight. Its slight occasional falls, whose precipices
would not diversify the landscape, are celebrated by mist and spray, and attract
the traveler from far and near. From the remote interior, its current conducts
him by broad and easy steps, or by one gentler inclined plane, to the sea. Thus
by an early and constant yielding to the inequalities of the ground it secures

itself the easiest passage.

No domain of nature is quite closed to man at all times, and now we draw near to the empire of the fishes. Our feet glide swiftly over unfathomed depths, where in summer our line tempted the pout and perch, and where the stately pickerel lurked in the long corridors formed by the bulrushes. The deep, impenetrable marsh, where the heron waded and bittern squatted, is made pervious to our swift shoes, as if a thousand railroads had been made into it. With one impulse we are carried to the cabin of the muskrat, that earliest settler, and see him dart away under the transparent ice, like a furred fish, to his hole in the bank; and we glide rapidly over meadows where lately 'the mower whet his scythe,' through beds of frozen cranberries mixed with meadowgrass. We skate near to where the blackbird, the pewee, and the kingbird hung their nests over the water, and the hornets builded from the maple in the swamp, How many gay warblers, following the sun, have radiated from this nest of silver birch and thistledown! On the swamp's outer edge was hung the supermarine village, where no foot penetrated. In this hollow tree the wood duck reared her brood, and slid away each day to forage in yonder fen.

In winter, nature is a cabinet of curiosities, full of dried specimens, in their natural order and position. The meadows and forests are a *hortus siccus*. The leaves and grasses stand perfectly pressed by the air without screw or gum, and the birds' nests are not hung on an artificial twig, but where they builded them. We go about dry-shod to inspect the summer's work in the rank swamp, and see what a growth have got the alders, the willows, and the maples; testifying to how many warm suns, and fertilizing dews and showers. See what strides their boughs took in the luxuriant summer—and anon these dormant buds will carry them onward and upward another span into the heavens.

Occasionally we wade through fields of snow, under whose depths the river is lost for many rods, to appear again to the right or left, where we least expected; still holding on its way underneath, with a faint, stertorous, rumbling sound, as if, like the bear and marmot, it too had hibernated, and we had followed its faint summer trail to where it earthed itself in snow and ice. At first we should have thought that rivers would be empty and dry in midwinter, or else frozen solid till the spring thawed them; but their volume is not diminished even, for only a superficial cold bridges their surfaces. The thousand springs which feed the lakes and streams are flowing still. The issues of a few surface springs only are closed, and they go to swell the deep reservoirs. Nature's wells are below the frost. The summer brooks are not filled with snow-water, nor does the mower quench his thirst with that alone. The streams are swollen when the snow melts in the spring, because nature's work has been delayed, the water being turned into ice and snow, whose particles are less smooth and round, and do not find their level so soon.

Far over the ice, between the hemlock woods and snow-clad hills, stands the pickerel-fisher, his lines set in some retired cove, like a Finlander, with his arms thrust into the pouches of his dreadnaught; with dull, snowy, fishy thoughts, himself a finless fish, separated a few inches from his race; dumb, erect, and made to be enveloped in clouds and snows, like the pines on shore. In these wild scenes, men stand about in the scenery, or move deliberately and heavily, having sacrificed the sprightliness and vivacity of towns to the dumb sobriety of nature. He does not make the scenery less wild, more than the jays and muskrats, but stands there as a part of it, as the natives are represented in the voyages of early navigators, at Nootka Sound, and on the Northwest coast, with their furs about them, before they were tempted to loquacity by a scrap of iron. He belongs to the natural family of man, and is planted deeper in nature and has more root than the inhabitants of towns. Go to him, ask what luck, and you will learn that he too is a worshiper of the unseen. Hear with what sincere deference and waving gesture in his tone he speaks of the lake pickerel which he has never seen, his primitive and ideal race of pickerel. He is connected with the shore still, as by a fishline, and yet remembers the season when he took fish through the ice on the pond, while the peas were up in his garden at home.

But now, while we have loitered, the clouds have gathered again, and a few straggling snowflakes are beginning to descend. Faster and faster they fall, shutting out the distant objects from sight. The snow falls on every wood and field, and no crevice is forgotten; by the river and the pond, on the hill and in the valley. Quadrupeds are confined to their coverts and the birds sit upon their perches this peaceful hour. There is not so much sound as in fair weather, but silently and gradually every slope, and the gray walls and fences, and the polished ice, and the sere leaves, which were not buried before, are concealed, and the tracks of men and beasts are lost. With so little effort does nature reassert her rule and blot out the traces of men. Hear how Homer has described the same: "The snowflakes fall thick and fast on a winter's day. The winds are lulled, and the snow falls incessant, covering the tops of the mountains, and the hills, and the plains where the lotus tree grows, and the cultivated fields, and they are falling by the inlets and shores of the foaming sea, but are silently dissolved by the waves." The snow levels all things, and infolds them deeper in the bosom of nature, as, in the slow summer, vegetation creeps up to the entablature of the temple, and the turrets of the castle, and helps her to prevail over art.

The surly night wind rustles through the wood, and warns us to retrace our steps, while the sun goes down behind the thickening storm, and birds seek their roosts, and cattle their stalls.

> "Drooping the labr'er ox
> Stands covered o'er with snow, and *now* demands
> The fruit of all his toil."

Though winter is represented in the almanac as an old man, facing the wind and sleet, and drawing his cloak about him, we rather think of him as a merry woodchopper, and warm-blooded youth, as blithe as summer. The unexplored grandeur of the storm keeps up the spirits of the traveler. It does not trifle with us, but has a sweet earnestness. In winter we lead a more inward life. Our hearts are warm and cheery, like cottages under drifts, whose windows and doors are half concealed, but from whose chimneys the smoke cheerfully ascends. The imprisoning drifts increase the sense of comfort which the house affords, and in the coldest days we are content to sit over the hearth and see the sky through the chimney-top, enjoying the quiet and serene life that may be had in a warm corner by the chimney-side, or feeling our pulse by listening to the low of cattle in the street, or the sound of the flail in distant barns all the long afternoon. No doubt a skillful physician could determine our health by observing how these simple and natural sounds affected us. We enjoy now, not an Oriental, but a Boreal leisure, around warm stoves and fireplaces, and watch the shadow of motes in the sunbeams.

Sometimes our fate grows too homely and familiarly serious ever to be cruel. Consider how for three months the human destiny is wrapped in furs. The good Hebrew Revelation takes no cognizance of all this cheerful snow. Is there no religion for the temperate and frigid zones? We know of no scripture which records the pure benignity of the gods on a New England winter night. Their praises have never been sung, only their wrath deprecated. The best scripture, after all, records but a meager faith. Its saints live reserved and austere. Let a brave, devout man spend the year in the woods of Maine or Labrador, and see if the Hebrew Scriptures speak adequately to his condition and experience, from the setting in of winter to the breaking up of the ice.

Now commences the long winter evening around the farmer's hearth, when the thoughts of the indwellers travel far abroad, and men are by nature and necessity charitable and liberal to all creatures. Now is the happy resistance to cold, when the farmer reaps his reward, and thinks of his preparedness for winter, and, through the glittering panes, sees with equanimity 'the mansion of the northern bear,' for now the storm is over,

> "The full ethereal round,
> Infinite worlds disclosing to the view,
> Shines out intensely keen; and all one cope
> Of starry glitter glows from pole to pole."

William Blake
WITH HAPPINESS STRETCHD
ACROSS THE HILLS

[To Thomas Butts, 22 November 1802]

With happiness stretchd across the hills
In a cloud that dewy sweetness distills
With a blue sky spread over with wings
And a mild sun that mounts & sings
With trees & fields full of Fairy elves
And little devils who fight for themselves
Remembring the Verses that Hayley sung
When my heart knockd against the root of my tongue
With Angels planted in Hawthorn bowers
And God himself in the passing hours
With Silver Angels across my way
And Golden Demons that none can stay
With my Father hovering upon the wind
And my Brother Robert just behind
And my Brother John the evil one
In a black cloud making his mone
Tho dead they appear upon my path
Notwithstanding my terrible wrath
They beg they intreat they drop their tears
Filld full of hopes filld full of fears
With a thousand Angels upon the Wind
Pouring disconsolate from behind
To drive them off & before my way
A frowning Thistle implores my stay
What to others a trifle appears

Fills me full of smiles or tears
For double the vision my Eyes do see
And a double vision is always with me
With my inward Eye 'tis an old Man grey
With my outward a Thistle across my way
"If thou goest back the thistle said
Thou art to endless woe betrayd
For here does Theotormon lower
And here is Enitharmons bower
And Los the terrible thus hath sworn
Because thou backward dost return
Poverty Envy old age & fear
Shall bring thy Wife upon a bier
And Butts shall give what Fuseli gave
A dark black Rock & a gloomy Cave"

I struck the Thistle with my foot
And broke him up from his delving root
"Must the duties of life each other cross"
"Must every joy be dung & dross"
'Must my dear Butts feel cold neglect"
"Because I give Hayley his due respect"
"Must Flaxman look upon me as wild"
"And all my friends be with doubts beguild"
"Must my Wife live in my Sisters bane"
"Or my sister survive on my Loves pain"
"The curses of Los the terrible shade"
"And his dismal terrors make me afraid"

So I spoke & struck in my wrath
The old man weltering upon my path
Then Los appeard in all his power
In the Sun he appeard descending before
My face in fierce flames in my double sight
Twas outward a Sun: inward Los in his might

"My hands are labourd day & night"
"And Ease comes never in my sight"
"My Wife has no indulgence given"
"Except what comes to her from heaven"
"We eat little we drink less"
"This Earth breeds not our happiness"
"Another Sun feeds our lifes streams"
"We are not warmed with thy beams"
"Thou measurest not the Time to me"
"Nor yet the Space that I do see"
"My Mind is not with thy light arrayd"
"Thy terrors shall not make me afraid"

When I had my Defiance given
The Sun stood trembling in heaven
The Moon that glowd remote below
Became leprous & white as snow
And every Soul of men on the Earth
Felt affliction & sorrow & sickness & dearth
Los flamd in my path & the Sun was hot
With the bows of my Mind & the Arrows of Thought
My bowstring fierce with Ardour breathes
My arrows glow in their golden sheaves
My brothers & father march before
The heavens drop with human gore

Now I a fourfold vision see
And a fourfold vision is given to me
Tis fourfold in my supreme delight
And three fold in soft Beulahs night
And twofold Always. May God us keep
From Single vision & Newtons sleep

Robert Frost
THE WOOD-PILE

Out walking in the frozen swamp one gray day
I paused and said, "I will turn back from here.
No, I will go on farther—and we shall see."
The hard snow held me, save where now and then
One foot went through. The view was all in lines
Straight up and down of tall slim trees
Too much alike to mark or name a place by
So as to say for certain I was here
Or somewhere else: I was just far from home.
A small bird flew before me. He was careful
To put a tree between us when he lighted,
And say no word to tell me who he was
Who was so foolish as to think what *he* thought.
He thought that I was after him for a feather—
The white one in his tail; like one who takes
Everything said as personal to himself.
One flight out sideways would have undeceived him.
And then there was a pile of wood for which
I forgot him and let his little fear
Carry him off the way I might have gone,
Without so much as wishing him good-night.
He went behind it to make his last stand.
It was a cord of maple, cut and split
And piled—and measured, four by four by eight.
And not another like it could I see.
No runner tracks in this year's snow looped near it.
And it was older sure than this year's cutting,
Or even last year's or the year's before.

The wood was gray and the bark warping off it
And the pile somewhat sunken. Clematis
Had wound strings round and round it like a bundle.
What held it though on one side was a tree
Still growing, and on one a stake and prop,
These latter about to fall. I thought that only
Someone who lived in turning to fresh tasks
Could so forget his handiwork on which
He spent himself, the labor of his ax,
And leave it there far from a useful fireplace
To warm the frozen swamp as best it could
With the slow smokeless burning of decay.

Natalia Ginzburg
WORN-OUT SHOES

My shoes are worn out, and the friend I live with at the moment also has worn-out shoes. When we are together we often talk about shoes. If I talk about the time when I shall be an old, famous writer, she immediately asks me "What shoes will you wear?" Then I say I shall have shoes made of green suede with a big gold buckle on one side.

I belong to a family in which everyone has sound, solid shoes. My mother possessed so many pairs of shoes that she even had to have a little wardrobe made especially for them. Whenever I visit them they utter cries of indignation and sorrow at the sight of my shoes. But I know that it is possible to live even with worn-out shoes. During the German occupation I was alone here in Rome, and I only had one pair of shoes. If I had taken them to the cobbler's I would have had to stay in bed for two or three days, and in my situation that was impossible. So I continued to wear them and when—on top of everything else—it rained, I felt them gradually falling apart, becoming soft and shapeless, and I felt the coldness of the pavement beneath the soles of my feet. This is why I still wear worn-out shoes, because I remember that particular pair and compared with them my present shoes don't seem too bad; besides, if I have money I would rather spend it on something else as shoes don't seem to me to be very essential things. When I was young I was always surrounded by tender, solicitous affection and I was spoilt, but that year when I was here in Rome I was alone for the first time and this is why I like Rome so much— even though it is full of history for me, full of terrible memories and very few hours of happiness. My friend also has worn-out shoes, and this is why we get on well together. My friend has no one to reproach her about the shoes she wears, she has only a brother who lives in the country and goes around in hunting boots. She and I know what happens when it rains, and your bare legs get soaked and the water comes into your shoes, so that there is a slight sound—a kind of soft squelch—at every step.

My friend has a pale, masculine face and when she smokes she uses a black cigarette-holder. The first time that I saw her, seated at a table, with her tortoise-shell rimmed spectacles and her mysterious, haughty face, with the black cigarette-holder gripped between her teeth, I thought she looked like a Chinese general. At that time I did not know that she had worn-out shoes. I discovered this later.

We have only known each other a few months, but it seems as many years. My friend has no children; I, on the other hand, do have children and to her this is odd. She has never seen them, except in a photograph, because they live in the provinces with my mother, and this too—that she has never seen my children—is very odd for both of us. In one sense she has no problems, she can give in to the temptation to let her life go to pieces; I, on the other hand, cannot. So, my children live with my mother and so far they do not have worn-out shoes. But what kind of men will they be? I mean, what kind of shoes will they have when they are men? What road will they choose to walk down? Will they decide to give up everything that is pleasant but not necessary, or will they affirm that everything is necessary and that men have the right to wear sound, solid shoes on their feet?

My friend and I talk about this a great deal, and about how the world will be when I am an old, famous writer and she will go wandering through the world with a rucksack on her back like an old Chinese general, and my children will go along their road with sound, solid shoes and the firm step of someone who doesn't give up, or with worn-out shoes and the slow, dragging step of someone who understands what is not necessary.

Sometimes we arrange marriages between my children and the children of her brother, the one who goes around the country in hunting boots. We talk like this until the small hours of the night and drink black, bitter tea. We have a mattress and a bed, and every evening we toss up for which of the two of us shall sleep in the bed. When we get up in the morning our worn-out shoes are waiting for us on the rug.

Now and again my friend says that she is fed up with working and wants to let her life go to pieces. She wants to shut herself in some filthy bar and drink all her savings, or she will just stay in bed and think of nothing and leave everything to drift, and let them come and cut off the gas and the light. She says she will do it when I leave. Because our shared life will not last much longer; soon I shall leave and return to my mother and children and be in a house where no one is allowed to have worn-out shoes. My mother will take me in hand; she will stop me using pins instead of buttons and writing till the small hours. And, in my turn, I shall take my children in hand and overcome the temptation to let my life go to pieces. I shall become serious and motherly, as always happens when I am with them, a different person from the one I am now—a person my friend does not know at all.

I shall watch the clock and keep track of time, I shall be cautious and wary about everything and I shall take care that my children's feet are always warm and dry, as I know that they must be if it is at all possible—at least during infancy. And perhaps even for learning to walk in worn-out shoes, it is as well to have dry, warm feet when we are children.

Eudora Welty
A WORN PATH

It was December—a bright frozen day in the early morning. Far out in the country there was an old Negro woman with her head tied in a red rag, coming along a path through the pinewoods. Her name was Phoenix Jackson. She was very old and small and she walked slowly in the dark pine shadows, moving a little from side to side in her steps, with the balanced heaviness and lightness of a pendulum in a grandfather clock. She carried a thin, small cane made from an umbrella, and with this she kept tapping the frozen earth in front of her. This made a grave and persistent noise in the still air, that seemed meditative like the chirping of a solitary little bird.

She wore a dark striped dress reaching down to her shoe tops, and an equally long apron of bleached sugar sacks, with a full pocket: all neat and tidy, but every time she took a step she might have fallen over her shoelaces, which dragged from her unlaced shoes. She looked straight ahead. Her eyes were blue with age. Her skin had a pattern all its own of numberless branching wrinkles and as though a whole little tree stood in the middle of her forehead, but a golden color ran underneath, and the two knobs of her cheeks were illumined by a yellow burning under the dark. Under the red rag her hair came down on her neck in the frailest of ringlets, still black, and with an odor like copper.

Now and then there was a quivering in the thicket. Old Phoenix said, "Out of my way, all you foxes, owls, beetles, jack rabbits, coons and wild animals! . . . Keep out from under these feet, little bob-whites. . . . Keep the big wild hogs out of my path. Don't let none of those come running my direction. I got a long way." Under her small black-freckled hand her cane, limber as a buggy whip, would switch at the brush as if to rouse up any hiding things.

On she went. The woods were deep and still. The sun made the pine needles almost too bright to look at, up where the wind rocked. The cones dropped as light as feathers. Down in the hollow was the mourning dove—it was not too late for him.

The path ran up a hill. "Seem like there is chains about my feet, time I get this far," she said, in the voice of argument old people keep to use with themselves. "Something always take a hold of me on this hill—pleads I should stay."

After she got to the top she turned and gave a full, severe look behind her where she had come. "Up through pines," she said at length. "Now down through oaks."

Her eyes opened their widest, and she started down gently. But before she got to the bottom of the hill a bush caught her dress.

Her fingers were busy and intent, but her skirts were full and long, so that before she could pull them free in one place they were caught in another. It was not possible to allow the dress to tear. "I in the thorny bush," she said. "Thorns, you doing your appointed work. Never want to let folks pass, no sir. Old eyes thought you was a pretty little *green* bush."

Finally, trembling all over, she stood free, and after a moment dared to stoop for her cane.

"Sun so high!" she cried, leaning back and looking, while the thick tears went over her eyes. "The time getting all gone here."

At the foot of this hill was a place where a log was laid across the creek.

"Now comes the trial," said Phoenix.

Putting her right foot out, she mounted the log and shut her eyes. Lifting her skirt, leveling her cane fiercely before her, like a festival figure in some parade, she began to march across. Then she opened her eyes and she was safe on the other side.

"I wasn't as old as I thought," she said.

But she sat down to rest. She spread her skirts on the bank around her and folded her hands over her knees. Up above her was a tree in a pearly cloud of mistletoe. She did not dare to close her eyes, and when a little boy brought her a plate with a slice of marble-cake on it she spoke to him. "That would be acceptable," she said. But when she went to take it there was just her own hand in the air.

So she left that tree, and had to go through a barbed-wire fence. There she had to creep and crawl, spreading her knees and stretching her fingers like a baby trying to climb the steps. But she talked loudly to herself: she could not let her dress be torn now, so late in the day, and she could not pay for having her arm or her leg sawed off if she got caught fast where she was.

At last she was safe through the fence and risen up out in the clearing. Big dead trees, like black men with one arm, were standing in the purple stalks of the withered cotton field. There sat a buzzard.

"Who you watching?"

In the furrow she made her way along.

"Glad this not the season for bulls," she said, looking sideways, "and the good Lord made his snakes to curl up and sleep in the winter. A pleasure I don't see no two-headed snake coming around that tree, where it come once. It took a while to get by him, back in the summer."

She passed through the old cotton and went into a field of dead corn. It whispered and shook and was taller than her head. "Through the maze now," she said, for there was no path.

Then there was something tall, black, and skinny there, moving before her.

At first she took it for a man. It could have been a man dancing in the field. But she stood still and listened, and it did not make a sound. It was as silent as a ghost.

"Ghost," she said sharply, "who be you the ghost of? For I have heard of nary death close by."

But there was no answer—only the ragged dancing in the wind.

She shut her eyes, reached out her hand, and touched a sleeve. She found a coat and inside that an emptiness, cold as ice.

"You scarecrow," she said. Her face lighted. "I ought to be shut up for good," she said with laughter. "My senses is gone. I too old. I the oldest people I ever know. Dance, old scarecrow," she said, "while I dancing with you."

She kicked her foot over the furrow, and with mouth drawn down, shook her head once or twice in a little strutting way. Some husks blew down and whirled in streamers about her skirts.

Then she went on, parting her way from side to side with the cane, through the whispering field. At last she came to the end, to a wagon track where the silver grass blew between the red ruts. The quail were walking around like pullets, seeming all dainty and unseen.

"Walk pretty," she said. "This the easy place. This the easy going."

She followed the track, swaying through the quiet bare fields, through the little strings of trees silver in their dead leaves, past cabins silver from weather, with the doors and windows boarded shut, all like old women under a spell sitting there. "I walking in their sleep," she said, nodding her head vigorously.

In a ravine she went where a spring was silently flowing through a hollow log. Old Phoenix bent and drank. "Sweet-gum makes the water sweet," she said, and drank more. "Nobody know who made this well, for it was here when I was born."

The track crossed a swampy part where the moss hung as white as lace from every limb. "Sleep on, alligators, and blow your bubbles." Then the track went into the road.

Deep, deep the road went down between the high green-colored banks. Overhead the live-oaks met, and it was as dark as a cave.

A black dog with a lolling tongue came up out of the weeds by the ditch. She was meditating, and not ready, and when he came at her she only hit him a little with her cane. Over she went in the ditch, like a little puff of milkweed.

Down there, her senses drifted away. A dream visited her, and she reached her hand up, but nothing reached down and gave her a pull. So she lay there and presently went to talking. "Old woman," she said to herself, "that black dog come up out of the weeds to stall you off, and now there he sitting on his fine tail, smiling at you."

A white man finally came along and found her—a hunter, a young man, with his dog on a chain.

"Well, Granny!" he laughed. "What are you doing there?"

"Lying on my back like a June-bug waiting to be turned over, mister," she said, reaching up her hand.

He lifted her up, gave her a swing in the air, and set her down. "Anything broken, Granny?"

"No sir, them old dead weeds is springy enough," said Phoenix, when she had got her breath. "I thank you for your trouble."

"Where do you live, Granny?" he asked, while the two dogs were growling at each other.

"Away back yonder, sir, behind the ridge. You can't even see it from here."

"On your way home?"

"No sir, I going to town."

"Why, that's too far! That's as far as I walk when I come out myself, and I get something for my trouble." He patted the stuffed bag he carried, and there hung down a little closed claw. It was one of the bob-whites, with its beak hooked bitterly to show it was dead. "Now you go on home, Granny!"

"I bound to go to town, mister," said Phoenix. "The time come around."

He gave another laugh, filling the whole landscape. "I know you old colored people! Wouldn't miss going to town to see Santa Claus!"

But something held old Phoenix very still. The deep lines in her face went into a fierce and different radiation. Without warning, she had seen with her own eyes a flashing nickel fall out of the man's pocket onto the ground.

"How old are you, Granny?" he was saying.

"There is no telling, mister," she said, "no telling."

Then she gave a little cry and clapped her hands and said, "Git on away from here, dog! Look! Look at that dog!" She laughed as if in admiration. "He ain't scared of nobody. He a big black dog." She whispered, "Sic him!"

"Watch me get rid of that cur," said the man. "Sic him, Pete! Sic him!"

Phoenix heard the dogs fighting, and heard the man running and throwing sticks. She even heard a gunshot. But she was slowly bending forward by that time, further and further forward, the lids stretched down over her eyes, as if she were doing this in her sleep. Her chin was lowered almost to her knees. The yellow palm of her hand came out from the fold of her apron. Her fingers slid down and along the ground under the piece of money with the grace and care they would have in lifting an egg from under a setting hen. Then she slowly straightened up, she stood erect, and the nickel was in her apron pocket. A bird flew by. Her lips moved. "God watching me the whole time. I come to stealing."

The man came back, and his own dog panted about them. "Well, I scared him off that time," he said, and then he laughed and lifted his gun and pointed it at Phoenix.

She stood straight and faced him.

"Doesn't the gun scare you?" he said, still pointing it.

"No, sir, I seen plenty go off closer by, in my day, and for less than what I done," she said, holding utterly still.

He smiled, and shouldered the gun. "Well, Granny," he said, "you must be a hundred years old, and scared of nothing. I'd give you a dime if I had any money with me. But you take my advice and stay home, and nothing will happen to you."

"I bound to go on my way, mister," said Phoenix. She inclined her head in the red rag. Then they went in different directions, but she could hear the gun shooting again and again over the hill.

She walked on. The shadows hung from the oak trees to the road like curtains. Then she smelled wood-smoke, and smelled the river, and she saw a steeple and the cabins on their steep steps. Dozens of little black children whirled around her. There ahead was Natchez shining. Bells were ringing. She walked on.

In the paved city it was Christmas time. There were red and green electric lights strung and criss-crossed everywhere, and all turned on in the daytime. Old Phoenix would have been lost if she had not distrusted her eyesight and depended on her feet to know where to take her.

She paused quietly on the sidewalk where people were passing by. A lady came along in the crowd, carrying an armful of red-, green- and silver-wrapped presents; she gave off perfume like the red roses in hot summer, and Phoenix stopped her.

"Please, missy, will you lace up my shoe?" She held up her foot.

"What do you want, Grandma?"

"See my shoe," said Phoenix. "Do all right for out in the country, but wouldn't look right to go in a big building."

"Stand still then, Grandma," said the lady. She put her packages down on the sidewalk beside her and laced and tied both shoes tightly.

"Can't lace 'em with a cane," said Phoenix. "Thank you, missy. I doesn't mind asking a nice lady to tie up my shoe, when I gets out on the street."

Moving slowly and from side to side, she went into the big building, and into a tower of steps, where she walked up and around and around until her feet knew to stop.

She entered a door, and there she saw nailed up on the wall the document that had been stamped with the gold seal and framed in the gold frame, which matched the dream that was hung up in her head.

"Here I be," she said. There was a fixed and ceremonial stiffness over her body.

"A charity case, I suppose," said an attendant who sat at the desk before her.

But Phoenix only looked above her head. There was sweat on her face, the wrinkles in her skin shone like a bright net.

"Speak up, Grandma," the woman said. "What's your name? We must have your history, you know. Have you been here before? What seems to be the trouble with you?"

Old Phoenix only gave a twitch to her face as if a fly were bothering her.

"Are you deaf?" cried the attendant.

But then the nurse came in.

"Oh, that's just old Aunt Phoenix," she said. "She doesn't come for herself—she has a little grandson. She makes these trips just as regular as clockwork. She lives away back off the Old Natchez Trace." She bent down. "Well, Aunt Phoenix, why don't you just take a seat? We won't keep you standing after your long trip." She pointed.

The old woman sat down, bolt upright in the chair.

"Now, how is the boy?" asked the nurse.

Old Phoenix did not speak.

"I said, how is the boy?"

But Phoenix only waited and stared straight ahead, her face very solemn and withdrawn into rigidity.

"Is his throat any better?" asked the nurse. "Aunt Phoenix, don't you hear me? Is your grandson's throat any better since the last time you came for the medicine?"

With her hands on her knees, the old woman waited, silent, erect and motionless, just as if she were in armor.

"You mustn't take up our time this way, Aunt Phoenix," the nurse said. "Tell us quickly about your grandson, and get it over. He isn't dead, is he?"

At last there came a flicker and then a flame of comprehension across her face, and she spoke.

"My grandson. It was my memory had left me. There I sat and forgot why I made my long trip."

"Forgot?" The nurse frowned. "After you came so far?"

Then Phoenix was like an old woman begging a dignified forgiveness for waking up frightened in the night. "I never did go to school, I was too old at the Surrender," she said in a soft voice. "I'm an old woman without an education. It was my memory fail me. My little grandson, he is just the same, and I forgot it in the coming."

"Throat never heals, does it?" said the nurse, speaking in a loud, sure voice to old Phoenix. By now she had a card with something written on it, a little list. "Yes. Swallowed lye. When was it?—January—two, three years ago—"

Phoenix spoke unasked now. "No, missy, he not dead, he just the same. Every little while his throat begin to close up again, and he not able to swallow. He not get his breath. He not able to help himself. So the time come around, and I go on another trip for the soothing medicine."

"All right. The doctor said as long as you came to get it, you could have it," said the nurse. "But it's an obstinate case."

"My little grandson, he sit up there in the house all wrapped up, waiting by himself," Phoenix went on. "We is the only two left in the world. He suffer and it don't seem to put him back at all. He got a sweet look. He going to last. He wear a little patch quilt and peep out holding his mouth open like a little bird. I remembers so plain now. I not going to forget him again, no, the whole enduring time. I could tell him from all the others in creation."

"All right." The nurse was trying to hush her now. She brought her a bottle of medicine. "Charity," she said, making a check mark in a book.

Old Phoenix held the bottle close to her eyes, and then carefully put it into her pocket.

"I thank you," she said.

"It's Christmas time, Grandma," said the attendant. "Could I give you a few pennies out of my purse?"

"Five pennies is a nickel," said Phoenix stiffly.

"Here's a nickel," said the attendant.

Phoenix rose carefully and held out her hand. She received the nickel and then fished the other nickel out of her pocket and laid it beside the new one. She stared at her palm closely, with her head on one side.

Then she gave a tap with her cane on the floor.

"This is what come to me to do," she said. "I going to the store and buy my child a little windmill they sells, made out of paper. He going to find it hard to believe there such a thing in the world. I'll march myself back where he waiting, holding it straight up in this hand."

She lifted her free hand, gave a little nod, turned around, and walked out of the doctor's office. Then her slow step began on the stairs, going down.

Guillaume Apollinaire
ZONE

Translated by Samuel Beckett

In the end you are weary of this ancient world

This morning the bridges are bleating Eiffel Tower oh herd

Weary of living in Roman antiquity and Greek

Here even the motor-cars look antique
Religion alone has stayed young religion
Has stayed simple like the hangars at Port Aviation

You alone in Europe Christianity are not ancient
The most modern European is you Pope Pius X
And you whom the windows watch shame restrains
From entering a church this morning and confessing your sins
You read the handbills the catalogues the singing posters
So much for poetry this morning and the prose is in the papers
Special editions full of crimes
Celebrities and other attractions for 25 centimes

This morning I saw a pretty street whose name is gone
Clean and shining clarion of the sun
Where from Monday morning to Saturday evening four times a day
Directors workers and beautiful shorthand typists go their way
And thrice in the morning the siren makes its moan
And a bell bays savagely coming up to noon
The inscriptions on walls and signs

The notices and plates squawk parrot-wise
I love the grace of this industrial street
In Paris between the Avenue des Ternes and the Rue Aumont-Thiéville

There it is the young street and you still but a small child
Your mother always dresses you in blue and white
You are very pious and with René Dalize your oldest crony
Nothing delights you more than church ceremony
It is nine at night the lowered gas burns blue you steal away
From the dormitory and all night in the college chapel pray
Whilst everlastingly the flaming glory of Christ
Wheels in adorable depths of amethyst
It is the fair lily that we all revere
It is the torch burning in the wind its auburn hair
It is the rosepale son of the mother of grief
It is the tree with the world's prayers ever in leaf
It is of honour and eternity the double beam
It is the six-branched star it is God
Who Friday dies and Sunday rises from the dead
It is Christ who better than airmen wings his flight
Holding the record of the world for height

Pupil Christ of the eye
Twentieth pupil of the centuries it is no novice
And changed into a bird this century soars like Jesus
The devils in the deeps look up and say they see a
Nimitation of Simon Magus in Judea
Craft by name by nature craft they cry
About the pretty flyer the angels fly
Enoch Elijah Apollonius of Tyana hover
With Icarus round the first airworthy ever
For those whom the Eucharist transports they now and then make way
Host-elevating priests ascending endlessly
The aeroplane alights at last with outstretched pinions
Then the sky is filled with swallows in their millions

The rooks come flocking the owls the hawks
Flamingoes from Africa and ibises and storks
The roc bird famed in song and story soars
With Adam's skull the first head in its clams
The eagle stoops screaming from heaven's verge
From America comes the little humming-bird
From China the long and supple
One-winged peehees that fly in couples
Behold the dove spirit without alloy
That ocellate peacock and lyre-bird convoy
The phoenix flame-devoured flame-revived
All with its ardent ash an instant hides
Leaving the perilous straits the sirens three
Divinely singing join the company
And eagle phoenix peehees fraternize
One and all with the machine that flies

Now you walk in Paris alone among the crowd
Herds of bellowing buses hemming you about
Anguish of love parching you within
As though you were never to be loved again
If you lived in olden times you would get you to a cloister
You are ashamed when you catch yourself at a paternoster
You are your own mocker and like hellfire your laughter crackles
Golden on your life's hearth fall the sparks of your laughter
It is a picture in a dark museum hung
And you sometimes go and contemplate it long

To-day you walk in Paris the women are blood-red
It was and would I could forget it was at beauty's ebb

From the midst of fervent flames Our Lady beheld me at Chartres
The blood of your Sacred Heart flooded me in Montmartre
I am sick with hearing the words of bliss
The love I endure is like a syphilis

And the image that possesses you and never leaves your side
In anguish and insomnia keeps you alive

Now you are on the Riviera among
The lemon-trees that flower all year long
With your friends you go for a sail on the sea
One is from Nice one from Menton and two from La Turbie
The polypuses in the depths fill us with horror
And in the seaweed fishes swim emblems of the Saviour

You are in an inn-garden near Prague
You feel perfectly happy a rose is on the table
And you observe instead of writing your story in prose
The chafer asleep in the heart of the rose
Appalled you see your image in the agates of Saint Vitus
That day you were fit to die with sadness
You look like Lazarus frantic in the daylight
The hands of the clock in the Jewish quarter go to left from right
And you too live slowly backwards
Climbing up to the Hradchin or listening as night falls
To Czech songs being sung in taverns

Here you are in Marseilles among the water-melons

Here you are in Coblentz at the Giant's Hostelry

Here you are in Rome under a Japanese medlar-tree

Here you are in Amsterdam with an ill-favoured maiden
You find her beautiful she is engaged to a student in Leyden
There they let their rooms in Latin cubicula locanda
I remember I spent three days there and as many in Gouda

You are in Paris with the examining magistrate
They clap you in gaol like a common reprobate

Grievous and joyous voyages you made
Before you knew what falsehood was and age
At twenty you suffered from love and at thirty again
My life was folly and my days in vain
You dare not look at your hands tears haunt my eyes
For you for her I love and all the old miseries

Weeping you watch the wretched emigrants
They believe in God they pray the women suckle their infants
They fill with their smell the station of Saint-Lazare
Like the wise men from the east they have faith in their star
They hope to prosper in the Argentine
And to come home having made their fortune
A family transports a red eiderdown as you your heart
An eiderdown as unreal as our dreams
Some go no further doss in the stews
Of the Rue des Rosiers or the Rue des Écouffes
Often in the streets I have seen them in the gloaming
Taking the air and like chessmen seldom moving
They are mostly Jews the wives wear wigs and in
The depths of shadowy dens bloodless sit on and on

You stand at the bar of a crapulous café
Drinking coffee at two sous a time in the midst of the unhappy

It is night you are in a restaurant it is superior

These women are decent enough they have their troubles however
All even the ugliest one have made their lovers suffer

She is a Jersey police-constable's daughter

Her hands I had not seen are chapped and hard

The seams of her belly go to my heart

To a poor harlot horribly laughing I humble my mouth

You are alone morning is at hand
In the streets the milkmen rattle their cans

Like a dark beauty night withdraws
Watchful Leah or Ferdine the false

And you drink this alcohol burning like your life
Your life that you drink like spirit of wine

You walk towards Auteuil you want to walk home and sleep
Among your fetishes from Guinea and the South Seas
Christs of another creed another guise
The lowly Christs of dim expectancies

Adieu Adieu

Sun corseless head

MORE LITERARY COMPANIONSHIP
FOR WALKERS

By now you have a sense of what we've learned about the literature of walking, and have probably found yourself wanting more of some things, and wondering why other things are not here. With that in mind, we'd like to offer some thoughts on what you might want to read next.

Some authors' writing seems saturated with walking, which appears again and again as their structuring principle, their favorite plot, scene, and symbol. In our collection you have already encountered some of these writers. Jane Austen, for instance, peppers her supposedly staid indoor fictions with adventurous walks, often by young women ignoring social convention, as Catherine Moreland does when she dashes alone through the streets of Bath in *Northanger Abbey,* or Elizabeth Bennet when she trudges cross-country to relieve her sister's illness in *Pride and Prejudice.* You already know Charles Dickens as the narrator of "Night Walks" who, despite the manic sunshine of the winter walk in *Martin Chuzzlewit,* more often darkens his walkers' paths with attendant scenes of murder, seduction, and, as Kim Taplin has noted, the death of the English countryside itself. Of Dickens's novels, in any of which you will find walking incidents, *The Old Curiosity Shop* is the one actually plotted as a walking "tour" (though a far from pleasurable one); and among his journalistic writings, *The Uncommercial Traveller* develops the walk through the nighttime city most fully.

But there are other fiction writers you will want to explore, if you haven't already noticed their interest in walking. Anne, Emily, and Charlotte Brontë, like Jane Austen, often create women walking more or less against the grain of their expected lives: Anne's Agnes Grey and Helen Huntingdon of *The Tenant of Wildfell Hall* ranging over the hills and by the sea, Emily's Nellie Dean on the path to Wuthering Heights, and Charlotte's Jane Eyre struggling across the moors toward her birthright. George Meredith's *The Egoist* and *Diana of the Crossways* offer us classically comic settings for the heroic walker crossing the landscape of English society. Thomas Hardy and James Joyce follow Dickens in their different ways, Hardy pressing on into the night of missed opportunity and failed understanding in *The Return of the Native,* or *Tess of the D'Urbervilles,* or *The Mayor of Casterbridge,* and Joyce taking Dublin as his London, perhaps most vividly in *Ulysses.* Virginia Woolf's *Mrs. Dalloway,* with its extraordinary Bond Street walk through the figurative shrapnel of post-World War I London, and E. M. Forster's *Howard's End,* with Leonard Bast's curiously affirming deflation of "RLS," are exemplary of the ways walking permeates these modernists' work.

For several of these fiction writers, the city clearly is the site of the most fruitful walking. You may also wish to trace the continental tradition of the flaneur who, as Walter Benjamin puts it, "goes botanizing on the asphalt," exploring the newly constructed urban spaces of the arcade and the department store. Benjamin's *Moscow Diaries* might be paired with the poetry and prose of his favorite, Charles Baudelaire, or with Fydor Dostoevsky's *Crime and Punishment,* in which Raskolnikov gives the flaneur a Nietzschean twist. This tradition reaches its climax in the work of the French surrealists, for whom walking through the modern city incarnates the spirit of daydreaming and free association. As Philip Lopate points out in his essay "The Pen on Foot: The Literature of Walking Around," novels like Louis Aragon's *Night Walker,* Philippe Soupault's *Last Nights of Paris,* and Andre Breton's *Nadja* all take walking in the city as their primary action, using it to explore the mysteries of chance, desire, and consciousness.

On the other hand, the continuing interest of British and American writers in "natural" or rural walks finds an answering voice in the work of many Chinese and Japanese writers. One translation of *Tao,* after all, is "the Way," and one possible reading of the *Tao Te Ching*'s opening line is "The way that can be walked is not the eternal Way." Any of the many translations of Lao-Tzu's *Tao Te Ching* will take you to the source of much Chinese and Japanese walking literature, but you might wish to try Stephen Addiss and Stanley Lombardo's graceful, spare translation. Taoism's persistent influence on the literature of walking cannot be separated from Buddhism's spiritualizing of the common, the everyday, and the "negative," and most particularly from Zen Buddhism and its poetic avatar, haiku. Any collection of Chinese or Japanese poetry would probably interest a reader of walking literature, but we particulary recommend the massive, beautiful 1975 anthology *Sunflower Splendor: Three Thousand Years of Chinese Poetry,* edited by Wu-chi Liu and Irving Yucheng Lo, and Robert Haas's 1994 edition of *The Essential Haiku: Versions of Bashō, Buson, and Issa.*

Among the British and American poets who constantly write about walking, we have already included William Wordsworth and John Clare, and some of their many heirs: Walt Whitman, Thomas Hardy, Robert Frost, Wendell Berry, A. R. Ammons, and Richard Long (whose work is only partly textual). And Gary Snyder must be counted one of the great poets of walking of any place or time, the heir and renewer of both Eastern and Western traditions of writing and walking. But you may not know that Dorothy Wordsworth's poems, though few in number, are as steeped in walking as her well-known journals (you can find them in Susan Levin's *Dorothy Wordsworth and Romanticism*); and you may not yet know Charlotte Smith, so influential in the early nineteenth century, whose often lyrical, sometimes gothic walking poems are now available again in an edition by Stuart Curran. Matthew Arnold is another regular nineteenth-century practitioner of the Wordsworthian recollective, meditative, often elegaic walking poem, as in "Thyrsis," "The Scholar-Gypsy" and "Stanzas from the Grande Chartreuse."

Besides the work of these and other writers with special affinities for walking, you can, of course, find literature about walking in every genre, by authors who do not take it as a constant theme, and in texts that may not use walking as a primary structure. Jeanie Dean's walk to London in Walter Scott's *The Heart of Mid-Lothian* anchors a long tale that may otherwise seem to treat pedestrian excursions incidentally;

Charles Brockden Brown's *Edgar Huntley: or, the Sleepwalker* is a performance Brown never repeats, but its wildly gothicized speculations on consciousness and reality, which seem a good two centuries ahead of its late-eighteenth-century publication, turn on the psychic difference—or is there any?—between walking and sleepwalking.

It is much more difficult to decide on similar examples of lyric poems that take walking as their occasion. Some favorites of ours we were unable to include here are T. S. Eliot's "Rhapsody on a Windy Night," Gwendolyn Brooks's "The Sundays of Satin-Legs Smith," Theodore Roethke's "The Far Field," Dylan Thomas's "Poem in October," W. H. Auden's "Walks," Edwin Denby's "Elegy—The Streets" Richard Wilbur's "Walking to Sleep," James Merrill's "An Urban Convalescence," Sylvia Plath's "Hardcastle Crags," Mary Oliver's "The Pinewoods," and Edward Hirsch's "Three Journeys" and "Dawn Walk." There are so many possibilities that we will stop here, with the fair certainty that you'll come across plenty of short walking poems no matter where you look. Our experience, well represented by Roger Gilbert's bibliographical "Epilogue" to his study of twentieth-century

American walking poetry, *Walks in the World,* is that such poems turn up with startling regularity.

The long poems that use walking to structure the whole or a significant part of the work include not only those by Gay, Cowper, William Wordsworth, and Barrett Browning excerpted here. Dante's *Inferno,* Richard Savage's *The Wanderer,* Goethe's *Faust,* W. Wordworth's *The Excursion,* Lord Byron's *Childe Harold,* Lord Tennyson's *In Memoriam: A. H. H.,* T. S. Eliot's *Four Quartets,* William Carlos Williams's *Paterson,* Wallace Stevens's "An Ordinary Evening in New Haven," Robert Penn Warren's *Audubon,* Allen Ginsberg's "Kaddish," Adrienne Rich's "Twenty-one Love Poems," and John Matthias's *A Gathering of Ways*—this list may serve to suggest the range of ways different poets, in different times, have reinterpreted walking to fit their notions of the life journey.

That particular notion of walking's potential to symbolize a wide variety of life-journeys, especially—the paradox is interesting—both that of the ordinary person and that of the unusually thoughtful one, also informs much philosophical and religious writing, represented here by Plato, Traherne, Bashō, Kan'ami, Rousseau, Blake, and Christina Rossetti. Other important examples from the British Christian tradition are the medieval mystery plays *Piers Plowman* and *Everyman*, and their literary descendent, John Bunyan's *Pilgrim's Progress.* If, as Sandra Gilbert and Susan Gubar have suggested, one then thinks of Charlotte Brontë's *Jane Eyre* as a revision of Bunyan, one has an interesting transit indeed.

In this anthology we have mostly avoided "real life" accounts of walking—travelogues, journals, diaries, letters, and the like—in favor of more obviously "fictionalized" versions of walking. But the distinction is never a clean one, nor should it be, we think. So Dorothy Wordsworth's Alfoxden and Grasmere journals, Thoreau's *The Maine Woods,* Emerson's journals, Keats's letters, Basho's *Narrow Road,* Clare's "Journey Out of Essex," and bits from Baudelaire and Benjamin are represented here. (For a satisfying companion to Keats, look for Carol Kyros Walker's recent book, *Walking North with Keats.*) Other works that might be mentioned in this context are the diaries of Francis Kilvert and Franz Kafka—rather seriously different in their perspectives and objects, but equally dependent on the walk as a means of observation. John James Audubon's multivolume *Ornithological Biography* and Vachel Lindsay's *Adventures While Preaching the Gospel of Beauty* make good companions for those who prefer the landscape of the American West, described in these two works at almost a century's distance from each other. Also of interest are those highly literary autobiographies that straddle the line between record and fiction, and the purpose of which is as much to recall a lost way of life as to recall a life, such as Alfred Kazin's *A Walker in the City,* Flora Thompson's *Lark Rise* trilogy, or Mary Russell Mitford's *Our Village.*

When, finally, we come to essays, we seem almost to have arrived at the heart of walking literature. It is rather odd that the essay should have such prominence, since the first essay that explicitly celebrates walking, William Hazlitt's "On Going a Journey" was published in 1821, and people have been writing about and through walking for much longer than that. Yet the anthologies of walking literature have always been full of such essays, sometimes to the exclusion of other genres. We chose Hazlitt, Thoreau, Dickens, Richard Jefferies, Woolf, and Linda Hogan, but we might have added Leslie Stephen, Robert Louis Stevenson, George Gissing, George Macaulay Trevelyan, Hilaire Belloc, John Burroughs, Annie Dillard, A. R. Ammons, Philip Lopate, Gary Snyder, Joyce Carol Oates, and more. It is in the essay, perhaps, that the senses long developing in poetry and fiction and philosophy, senses of walking as thought and meditation and memory, and as representative or individual life journeys, can be more plainly set out, examined, or exemplified. Here, caught up in the accelerating world Hazlitt felt pressing toward him, in the driven times Arnold knew had already overtaken him, we try, we "essay," to explain to ourselves what we believe about walking—a task no more capable of completion than this survey of walking literature.

Our suggestions for further reading reflect not only our own experience but also the work of many others interested in the literature of walking. In our lists of "Other Anthologies of Walking Literature" and "Literary and Historical Studies," below, you will find books that have influenced our selections, but that also can take you well beyond our choices. In the second of these lists, we have included only book-length works that take walking and walkers as a principal subject, omitting the many studies of transportation, rural or urban life, literary genre, etc., in which walking briefly figures.

We are only too aware of how unequal our small beginning is to the task of surveying walking literature. Missing from these pages are whole genres, peoples, philosophies, that would delight you. But we also know you will find your own way, a fuller way, from here.

OTHER ANTHOLOGIES OF WALKING LITERATURE

Belloc, Hillare, ed. *The Footpath Way.* 1911. Der Spaziergang: Ein Literarisches Lesebuch. Olms, 1992.

Goldmark, Pauline and Mary Hopkins, eds. *The Gypsy Trail: An Anthology for Campers.* 1922.

Goodman, George. *The Lore of the Wanderer: An Open-Air Anthology.* 1920.

Graham, Stephen, ed. *The Gentle Art of Tramping.* New York: D. Appleton & Co., 1926.

Mitchell, Edwin Valentine, ed. *The Pleasures of Walking.* 1934.

Sidgwick, A. H., ed. *Walking Essays.* London: Edward Arnold, 1912.

Sussman, Aaron and Ruth Goode, eds. *The Magic of Walking.* New York: Simon and Schuster, 1967.

Trent, George D., ed. *The Gentle Art of Walking.* New York: Arno–Random House, 1971.

Zochert, Donald, ed. *Walking in America.* New York: Alfred A. Knopf, 1974.

LITERARY AND HISTORICAL STUDIES

Barta, Peter I., *Bely, Joyce, and Doblin: Peripatetics in the City Novel.* Gainesville: University of Florida Press, 1996.

Benjamin, Walter. *Charles Baudelaire: A Lyric Poet in the Era of High Capitalism.* Trans. Harry Zohn. London: New Left Books, 1973.

Brand, Dana. *The Spectator and the City in Nineteenth-Century American Literature.* Cambridge, U.K.: Cambridge University Press, 1991.

Bushnell, Nelson S. *A Walk After John Keats.* New York: Farrar & Rineholt, 1936.

Cohen, Margaret. *Profane Illumination: Walter Benjamin and the Paris of Surrealist Revolution.* University of California Press, 1993.

Cummings, John. *Runners and Walkers: A Nineteenth-Century Sports Chronicle.* Chicago: Regnery Gateway, 1981.

Elder, John. *Imagining the Earth: Poetry and the Vision of Nature.* Urbana and Chicago: University of Illlinois Press, 1985.

Chambers, Ross. *Loiterature.* Lincoln: University of Nebraska Press, 1999.

Gleber, Anke. *The Art of Taking a Walk: Flanerie, Literature and Film in Weimar Culture.* Princeton, NJ: Princeton University Press, 1999.

Gilbert, Roger. *Walks in the World: Representation and Experience in Modern American Poetry.* Princeton, NJ: Princeton University Press, 1991.

Holmes, Richard. *Footsteps: Adventures of a Romantic Biographer.* New York: Viking, 1985.

Jarvis, Robin. *Romantic Writing and Pedestrian Travel.* Houndsmill and London: Macmillian; New York: St. Martins, 1997.

Jusserand, J. J. *English Wayfaring Life in the Middle Ages.* London: T. Fisher Unwin, 1888.

Langan, Celeste. *Romantic Vagrancy: Wordsworth and the Simulation of Freedom.* Cambridge: Cambridge University Press, 1996.

Marples, Morris. *Shanks's Pony: A Study of Walking.* London: J.M. Dent & Sons, 1959.

Nord, Deborah Epstein. *Walking the Victorian Streets: Women, Representation and the City.* Ithaca and New York: Cornell University Press, 1995.

Robinson, Jeffrey. *The Walk: Notes on a Romantic Image.* Norman: University of Oklahoma Press, 1989.

Strickland, Ron. *Shank's Mare: A Compendium of Remarkable Walks.* New York: Paragon House, 1988.

Taplin, Kim. *The English Path.* Woodbridge, Suffolk: The Boydell Press, 1979.

Wallace, Anne D. *Walking, Literature, and English Culture: The Origin and Uses of Peripatetic in the Nineteenth Century.* Oxford: Clarendon, 1993.

ACKNOWLEDGMENTS

"Ask for Nothing" from *The Simple Truth* by Philip Levine. Copyright 1994 by Philip Levine. Reprinted by permission of Alfred A. Knopf Inc.

"Bread-and-Butter" from *Tesserae* by John Hollander. Copyright 1993 by John Hollander. Reprinted by permission of Alfred A. Knopf Inc.

"Corsons Inlet," copyright 1963 by A. R. Ammons, from *Collected Poems 1951–1971* by A. R. Ammons. Reprinted by permission of W. W. Norton & Company, Inc.

"Crowds, by Charles Baudelaire, translated by Louis Varese, from *Paris Spleen,* copyright 1947 by New Directions Publishing Corp. Reprinted by permission of New Directions Publishing Corp.

"The Day Lady Died" by Frank O'Hara. Copyright 1964. Reprinted from *Lunch Poems* by permission of City Lights Books.

"The End of March" from *The Complete Poems 1927–1979* by Elizabeth Bishop. Copyright 1979, 1983 by Alice Helen Methfessel. Reprinted by permission of Farrar, Straus and Giroux, LLC.

"A Four Day Walk" by Richard Long. Published in *Richard Long,* ed. R. H. Fuchs, London and New York: Thames and Hudson / Solomon Guggenheim, copyright 1986. Reprinted by permission of the author.

"Hashish in Marseilles" from *Reflections: Essays, Aphorisms, Autobiographical Writings* by Walter Benjamin, English translation copyright 1978 by Harcourt, Inc., reprinted by permission of the publisher.

"Journeying by Stream: Following Chin-Chu Torrent I Cross the Mountains" by Hsieh Ling-Yun, translated by Francis Westbrook. Copyright 1975. Reprinted from *Sunflower Splendor: Three Thousand Years of Chinese Poetry,* ed. Wu-chi Liu and Irving Yucheng Lo, by permission of Wu-chi Liu.

"La Junta" by Simon J. Ortiz. Permission granted by Simon J. Ortiz. Published originally in *From Sand Creek*, The University of Arizona Press, Tucson, Arizona, 2000.

"A Little Ramble" from *Selected Stories* by Robert Walser, trans. by Christopher Middleton. Translation copyright 1982 by Farrar, Straus & Giroux, Inc. Reprinted by permission of Farrar, Straus and Giroux.

"a long walk, from *Series* by Robert Grenier, published by This Press. Copyright 1978. Reprinted by permission of the author.

Narrow Road to the Interior by Basho, translated by Sam Hamill, 1991. Reprinted by arrangement with Shambhala Publications, Inc., Boston.

"Ode 17" by Petrarch, in Petrarch's *Canzoniere* translated by Mark Musa. Reprinted by permission of Indiana University Press.

"The Ones Who Walk Away from Omelas" by Ursula K. LeGuin. Copyright 1973. Reprinted by permission of Ursula K. LeGuin and Virginia Kidd Agency, Inc.

"Orpheus, Eurydice, and Hermes" by Rainer Maria Rilke from *Imitations* by Robert Lowell. Copyright 1959 by Robert Lowell. Copyright renewed 1987 by Harriet, Sheridan, and Caroline Lowell. Reprinted by permission of Farrar, Straus & Giroux, LLC.

"The Pedestrian" by Ray Bradbury. Copyright 1952. Reprinted from *Golden Apples of the Sun* by permission of Don Congdon Associates.

"Returning" from *The Wheel* by Wendell Berry. Copyright 1982 by Wendell Berry. Reprinted by permission of North Point Press, a division of Farrar, Straus and Giroux.

"Second Walk" from *Reveries of the Solitary Walker* by Jean Jacques Rousseau, translated by Charles E. Butterworth. Copyright 1979. Reprinted by permission of New York University Press.

"Setting Out" from *The Wheel* by Wendell Berry. Copyright 1982 by Wendell Berry. Reprinted by permission of North Point Press, a division of Farrar, Straus & Giroux.

"Sotoba Komachi" by Kan'ami Kiyotsugu, translated by Sam Houston Brock, from *Anthology of Japanese Literature from the Earliest Era to the Mid-Nineteenth Century,* edited by Donald Keene. Copyright 1955 by Grove Press, Inc. Used by permission of Grove/Atlantic, Inc.

"A Step Away from Them" by Frank O'Hara. Copyright 1964. Reprinted from *Lunch Poems* by permission of City Lights Books.

"Stepping Westward," by Denise Levertov, from *Poems 1960-1967,* copyright 1966 by Denise Levertov. Reprinted by permission of New Directions Publishing Corp.

"Street Haunting" from *The Death of the Moth and Other Essays* by Virginia Woolf, copyright 1942 by Harcourt, Inc. and renewed 1970 by Marjorie T. Parsons, Executrix, reprinted by permission of the publisher.

"The Sudden Walk" from *Franz Kafka: The Complete Stories* by Franz Kafka. Copyright 1971 by Schocken Books. Reprinted by permission of Schocken Books, distributed by Pantheon Books, a division of Random House Inc.

"Sunday Walks in the Suburbs" copyright 1977 by Marie Syrkin Reznikoff. Reprinted from *Poems 1918-1975: The Complete Poems of Charles Reznikoff* with the permission of Black Sparrow Press.

"A Supermarket in California" from *Collected Poems 1947-1980* by Allen Ginsberg. Copyright 1955 by Allen Ginsberg. Copyright Renewed. Reprinted by permission of HarperCollins Publishers, Inc.

"There Is a Way to Walk on Water" by Patiann Rogers was published in *Firekeeper: New and Selected Poems* (Milkweed, 1994). Copyright 1994 by Patiann Rogers. Reprinted with permission from Milkweed Editions.

"Upper Broadway" from *The Fact of a Doorframe: Poems Selected and New, 1950-1984* by Adrienne Rich. Copyright 1984 by Adrienne Rich. Copyright 1975, 1978 by W.W. Norton & Company, Inc. Copyright 1981 by Adrienne Rich. Reprinted by permission of the author and W.W. Norton & Company, Inc.

"The Useless Vigil" by Gabriela Mistral from *A Gabriela Mistral Reader*. Translated by Maria Giachetti. Copyright 1993 by White Pine Press, reprinted by permission of the publisher.

"A Walk" by Gary Snyder, from *The Back Country,* copyright 1968 by Gary Snyder. Reprinted by permission of New Directions Publishing Corp.

"The Walk" reprinted here on pages 294-300, from *Rain Darling* by Merle Collins, first published by The Women's Press Ltd., 1990, 34 Great Sutton Street, London EC1V 0LQ, is used by permission of The Women's Press Ltd.

"Walking," from *The Journey Home* by Edward Abbey. Copyright 1977 by Edward Abbey. Used by permission of Dutton, a division of Penguin Putnam Inc.

"Walking," copyright 1990 by Linda Hogan, from *Dwellings: A Spiritual History of the Living World* by Linda Hogan. Reprinted by permission of W. W. Norton & Company, Inc.

"Walking Around" by Pablo Neruda, translated by Robert Bly. Reprinted from *Neruda and Vallejo: Selected Poems,* edited by Robert Bly, Beacon Press, Boston, 1993. Copyright 1993 Robert Bly. Reprinted with his permission.

"Walking Our Boundaries," from *The Black Unicorn* by Audre Lorde. Copyright 1978 by Audre Lorde. Reprinted by permission of W. W. Norton & Company, Inc.

"Worn-Out Shoes" from *Little Virtues,* by Natalia Ginzburg, translated by Dick Davis. Copyright 1985. Reprinted by permission of Carcanet Press.

"A Worn Path" from *A Curtain of Green and Other Stories,* copyright 1941 and renewed 1969 by Eudora Welty, reprinted by permission of Harcourt, Inc.

"Zone" by Guillaume Apollinaire, translated by Samuel Beckett, from *Collected Poems in English and French* by Samuel Beckett. Copyright 1977 by Samuel Beckett. Used by permission of Grove/Atlantic, Inc.

THEMATIC INDEX

SOCIETY—from *Persuasion,* from *Reveries of a Solitary Walker*, "Song of the Open Road," "A Step Away from Them," "Street Haunting," "A Supermarket in California," "Of Walking the Streets at Night," "Walking Around"

SPIRITUALITY—from *Aurora Leigh,* "The Hills are tipped with sunshine," "Hurrahing in Harvest," "I Walk'd the Other Day," from *The Narrow Road to the Interior,* from *The Prelude,* "Regeneration," "Resolution and Independence," "Returning," from *Reveries of a Solitary Walker,* "Song of the Open Road," "Sotoba Komachi," "Stepping Westward" (Levertov), "Stepping Westward" (Wordsworth), "There Is a Way to Walk on Water," "This Lime-Tree Bower My Prison," "The Useless Vigil," "A Walk" (Rilke), "Walking" (Traherne), "The Wild Common," "With Happiness Stretchd across the Hills," "Zone"

SUBURBS AND TOWNS—"La Junta," "Looking for Signs," "Sunday Walks in the Suburbs"

WATER—from *The Maine Woods,* "The Tarn," "There is a Way to Walk on Water," "A Winter Walk"

Sports literature from BREAKAWAY BOOKS